Must Have Been
SOMETHING I ATE

The simple connection between what
you eat and how you look and feel.

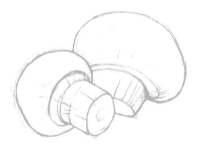

by: Peggy Kotsopoulos

Published by Oceanside Publishing Ink – 33 – 1833 Coast Meridian Road, Port Coquitlam BC V3C 6G5

This publication contains the opinion and ideas of its author and is designed to provide useful advice in regards to the subject matter covered for information purposes only. This publication is sold with the understanding that neither the author nor the publisher is engaged in rendering health advice or professional services in this publication. The publication is not intended to provide a basis for action in particular circumstances without consideration by a competent professional.

The information contained in this publication cannot replace or substitute for the services of trained professionals in the medical field. You should not act upon any of the information offered or provided within or through this publication without seeking professional advice. In particular, you should regularly consult a doctor in all matters relating to physical or mental health, particularly concerning any symptoms that may require diagnosis or medical attention.

Printed in Canada.
ISBN: 9780986548819

Photography: Jalani Morgan & Shawn Taylor
Food stylist: Peggy Kotsopoulos & Lawren Moneta
Illustration: Sooh Yun Jung
Graphic Design: Any Widjaja
Creative Direction: John Edmonds

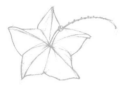

To my parents, for their unrelenting support, luv, belief in me
and not thinking that I'm totally nuts (more like a seed).

Table of Contents

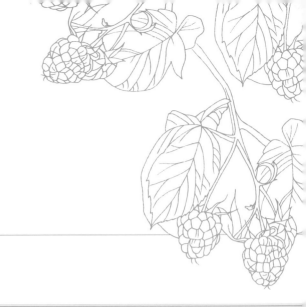

INTRODUCTION

We all know her — the perky, annoying chick who bounces into work in the morning. It's barely 7:30 a.m. and she's already finished a workout, walked her dog and made all her meals for the day. All this, and she still looks more put together than a cover model for Marc Jacobs. Seriously. What gives? Was she just born this way? Or does she know something we don't? Chances are, the secret to her success is actually very simple: it's something she ate. How you look and feel is a direct reflection of what you eat, and more importantly, what you assimilate. It affects pretty much everything, even things you wouldn't think of right away. Like, how about those tiny bumps on the back of your arm? The luster in your hair? Or the fact that you're just too damn tired to even *think* of having sex? The answer: yes, yes and, *hells yes* — all of these things have to do with what you eat. Food shapes the way you think, the way you process information, the clarity of your ideas and thoughts, your mood, your energy, your waist size, your libido, your skin and your metabolism. It's all about food! And that's a good thing, because who doesn't love food?

My passion for food started pretty much when I was born. I grew up in a Greek household, so I really had no choice. My life revolved around food! We weren't even done eating breakfast and my mother was already working on our next meal. But my *awareness* of how food made me feel began around the ripe old age of five. Even then, I knew if I ate a burger I would be sluggish and lethargic and wouldn't have the energy to play. Whereas if I ate a pint of strawberries, my face would get these vibrant little tingles and I'd be filled with energy. Gut instinct? Maybe. But about 10 years later, it all started to make even more sense.

At age 15, I was hit by a car that was going 80 km/hr on impact. I was broken into pieces. After hours upon hours of surgery and some serious complications, the doctors didn't think I would survive. But I knew I would. I believed this so firmly that I was out of the hospital in two and a half weeks. They called me "miracle child." But it wasn't a miracle. It was a choice I made while lying in that hospital bed, knowing I still had so much to live and to experience. And I wanted to live life to the fullest! This realization is what caused me to look long and hard at what I was eating and how food nourishes both the body and the soul. I remembered how those strawberries used to make my face tingle, and decided that's how I want to feel everyday! If we can make the choice to live in a state of optimal health — spiritually, emotionally and physically — why wouldn't we?

There is no excuse for not feeling your best. Yes, we can all have occasional off days where we'd rather hide under an oversized pair of aviators and a fedora hat and pretend real life is not out there waiting for us. But if you ever felt like you could use just a bit more energy and be less scatterbrained, or if you ever thought your skin could be brighter or you could stand to lose a few pounds, *you absolutely can*. Everyday. And it's not about major life changes like giving up your favourite things, running away to some boot camp or signing up for a reality TV weight-loss show. It's about making little changes that collectively can add up to something ginormous — completely transforming how you look and feel.

Because food affects, well, everything, I've divided this book into four sections — so you can quickly find the info that will help you the most. Chapters 1 through 5 take a look at the impact of what we eat on how we feel — how the right foods can boost our energy levels, reduce our stress levels, help us get more zzz's, rev up our sex drive and even combat depression. In chapters 6 through 9, I explain how food affects how we look, including combating those damn muffin tops and thunder thighs and which foods to eat to keep you looking smokin' hot. Chapters 10 to 12 explore the nutrients and foods that contribute to our immune and digestive health and even tips for combating psycho-chick PMS moments. Then at the end of the book I give you plenty of delish drink, app, soup, salad, entree and dessert recipes to put everything you've learned into practice, so you don't have to think so much.

Before we bite right into how food affects our minds and bodies, here are some key principles to remember:

YOU DON'T HAVE TO GIVE UP YOUR FAVOURITE FOODS
You know that ooie-gooie lasagna smothered in four types of cheese, baked to perfection in a chunky tomato sauce? Maybe not the best choice you could make. But that doesn't mean you have to give it up cold turkey forever. Imagine thinking you could never have a piece of lasagna for the rest of your life… ever. Chances are you'd suffer from some serious separation anxiety, be miserable and, in the end, fail. Don't go cold turkey on anything. Instead, start not by focusing on what you need to give up, just start by adding *more*. That's right, just add

more real, nutrient-dense whole foods to your diet and make small changes to the ingredients you use regularly. Start by using only half the cheese, replace the white refined noodles with brown rice noodles or even thinly sliced strips of eggplant or summer squash, and throw some spinach or sunflower sprouts into the mix. Or just have a small piece of the real thing and make the other half of your meal a peppery arugula salad topped with candied walnuts, freshly julienned pear and crispy sunflower sprouts sprinkled with creamy hemp seeds and a citrus olive oil drizzle. Doable? I think so. It's just about making those small changes. If you're at a fast food joint, nix the fries in your combo for a side salad. Try sprouted grain bread instead of whole wheat. Try kelp noodles instead of refined noodles in an Asian stir-fry. Trade in chocolate-covered peanuts for cocoa-kissed SaviSeeds. Top your meals with some sunflower sprouts. Once you start adding more goodness to your diet, you'll start feeling fabulous. Your energy will improve, your complexion will get clearer and your eyes will be brighter. As for the not-so-good stuff? You'll find that you don't really want it anymore, and it'll just naturally falls off your radar like that multi-coloured jersey dress that was so last season. And if you really want it — go ahead! Just be conscious of how you feel, and trust me, in time you'll be craving more of that arugula salad instead!

NOURISH YOUR SPIRIT

Sometimes it doesn't matter how well you eat. If you're in a bad headspace or are overly-stressed, you won't absorb nutrients, vitamins in your body will be depleted and antioxidants just can't keep up. I spent nearly 10 years in investments prior to delving wholeheartedly into my passion for nutrition. At the time, I thought I was the healthiest person around. I was a strict raw food vegan, worked out like a crazy chick and thought I was at the top of my game. Until I went down to the Hippocrates Health Institute in West Palm Beach and had a blood cell analysis done, that is. The results nearly killed me. Or, more accurately, I nearly killed me. *"What?"* I remember gasping. My antioxidant levels were at mere 27 per cent, when I thought they would be almost 100 per cent! At first, I didn't get it. I thought was doing everything right. That's when it hit me. I wasn't being true to myself. I was in job that didn't fulfill my purpose and I wasn't living in alignment with my own core values. My body was stressed. As I pursued my education in holistic nutrition, I made the connection. Although I didn't *think* I was stressed at the time, internally my body and mind were completely depleted. Only when I let go of everything that didn't truly matter to me did my health pick back up.

In order to achieve full health, we need to let go of things that have no meaning to us or do not serve the purpose we have for our lives. Once we let go of all that, we free up space in our own energy field, allowing that space to be filled with fulfillment, purpose, ultimate happiness and health! And all the goodness we consume from the food we eat will nourish us completely. If you're not there yet, don't worry — what you eat, as you will see in this book, may just help you get there. When you eat clean, it quiets your stomach. When you have quiet stomach, you have a quiet mind, and when you have a quiet mind, you can listen to your heart — and your heart speaks the truth.

PRACTICE MINDFUL EATING

I know, I know, we're all busy. Eating on the go — whether it's in the car, out the door, at the desk, or while running to the gym — is pretty much the norm. We all do it. But keep in mind that when you eat in such a hurried — and harried — manner, you're not in an optimal state to digest food and assimilate nutrients. As powerful as your body is, even superwoman can run into issues. Ask yourself why you are eating. Are you truly hungry, or just bored, stressed or low on energy? You need to make sure you're eating the right foods to get you going, and the right foods for *how* you feel. If you're tired, eat energy-boosting foods. If you're depressed, eat mood-boosting happy foods. If you're bored... then get your ass moving and hit the gym or go for a run! Food is energy. It nourishes our cells and our souls. Practice conscious eating. Know where your food is coming from and who is preparing your food. The reason why something is called "comfort" food doesn't have to be because it's high in calories and fat — it can be because it's made with love. So go ahead, enjoy a pint of strawberries and feel your face tingle!

REACH FOR REAL FOOD

If it came out of a box, bag or wrapper, chances are you're not giving yourself the absolute best nutrients your body deserves. Whenever possible, reach for real, fresh, whole food. Choosing mostly whole foods – ideally plant-based and unrefined – means that you are fueling your body with nutrient-rich, age-defying, disease-busting goodness. Shop the outside aisles of the grocery store or better yet hit the farmer's market. Choose whole foods in a wide-range of colours, flavours and textures to add variety and balance to your life.

And remember this doesn't mean you need to spend hours in the kitchen. Whole food eating can be as simple as grabbing an apple for a snack rather than that sugar-laden granola bar. Plus there are some great companies out there making strides in convenient natural health foods. Check out the Resources section on page 186 for details on my faves.

FOOD-MOOD CONNECTION

Explore the foodie connection to more energy, less stress, deeper sleep, better sex and elevated mood!

FOOD—MOOD CONNECTION

Our lives are surrounded by choice. Every second there's a choice to be made — do I stay in bed for an extra five minutes in the morning or get up right away? Do I go to the gym today or take another rest day? Should I make my lunch or buy my lunch? Although it may seem trivial, what you choose to *eat* each day is probably one of the most important decisions you make. What you eat directly impacts your thoughts, your actions, your mood and your psyche. What you eat is what you think, and what you think is what you become.

Many of us are emotional eaters. We tend to reach for comfort food in the hope it will fill an emotional void — which doesn't really work (although we may think it does). In this section, I'm going to show you the *right* type of emotional eating — mood foods! These foods will help get you out of your funk no matter how you're feeling. But before we begin, here's a look at how exactly food can affect your mind and mood.

HOW OUR MIND WORKS

Let's look how our brains work and how what we eat can impact more than just our waistlines. The brain is made up of about 100 billion neurons. Neurons are the brain's nerve cells that transmit information by electrical or chemical signaling. The chemical messengers that deliver communication from one neuron to another are called neurotransmitters. The space between neurons is called a synapse, which is where neurotransmitters swim to send and receive information. Here's the kicker: these neurotransmitters are partially responsible for our happiness, sadness, stress response, anger, energy, sex drive and overall mood and feeling. And they are made up of amino acids we get *through our food*. As well, certain

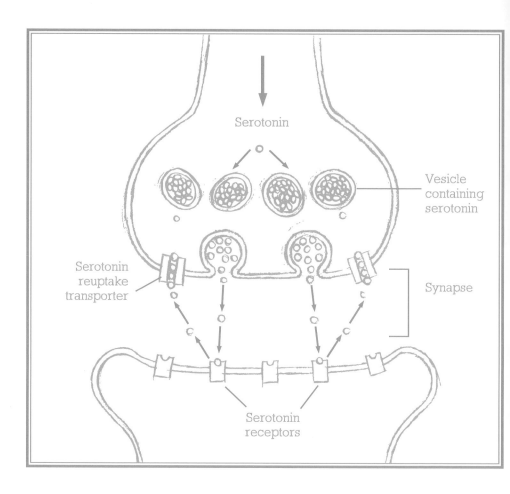

vitamins, minerals and nutrients are essential in the conversion of amino acids to neurotransmitters. Therefore, different foods have the ability to affect mood by altering the levels of neurotransmitters in the brain. Certain foods can either increase or suppress the messenger activity happening between the brain's billions of neurons.

Each neurotransmitter has its own specific receptor cell that it fits into and unlocks, kind of like a key, for communication to occur. In order for the message to get across, the neurotransmitter must bind onto a receptor cell, and one that fits.

How does this work? Think of the neurotransmitter as a plug, and the receptor cells as an electrical outlet. Now, imagine you're at the gym, just finished your workout, showered, and need to blow dry your hair. You go to plug in your blow dryer, and to your luck, you have tons of options. You can plug in by the big mirror, small mirror, full-length mirror, close to your friends, away from your friends, anywhere you want because there are outlets everywhere. So you're happy and you leave the gym with a fabulous blowout. But what if there are no electrical outlets, or the only ones left were a two-prong outlet, where your blow dryer had a three-prong plug, so it doesn't fit. You'd need to pack away that blow dryer and walk out with your mop-head wet hair wrapped under a hoodie, not feeling so glam.

The same thing can happen to neurotransmitters. Once they are released, if they don't bind onto a receptor cell, or if they don't fit, communication is lost.

Here are some examples of the various kinds of neurotransmitters and how they affect your mood:

Amino Acid	Neurotransmitter	Function
Tyrosine	Dopamine	Increases motivation, drive, sense of reward, pleasure.
Tryptophan	Serotonin (converts to melatonin)	Makes you happy! Boosts mood and fights depression.
	Melatonin	Helps you relax and sleep.
Glutamine	GABA	Calms and relaxes without stimulating.

The brain isn't the only organ that has receptors to neurotransmitters. Immune cells, blood cells and tissues also have receptors, and there's a lot of chit-chat going on between the brain, immune system, endocrine system and nervous system. Everything is connected and everything is affected by what you eat!

ENERGY

It's the crack of dawn, and the piercing sound of your alarm clock causes more pain than running around town in four-inch stilettos that are half a size too small. "Just five more minutes!" Or at least that's what you tell yourself as you hit snooze repeatedly for the next hour and a half. Then, when finally realizing you're oh-so-late, you fly out of bed, down half a litre of coffee and attempt to regain some consciousness and sensibility as you try to put yourself together and bolt out the door. Oops, didn't make the gym *again* this morning, but it's okay, you'll get there after work. Yep, that's what you'll do. After all, you're feeling pretty pumped at the moment from all the adrenaline kicking through your body as you race to get to your morning meeting on time. Albeit, you soon realize that high was extremely short-lived, and you now need to physically hold your eyelids open with the back of your pen as you sit through never-ending dialogue about… oh, it doesn't matter, you're not paying attention anyway.

So you pretend to take notes to force yourself from literally falling asleep in your seat. But it's not working. Your head is getting heavy, you have no clue what anyone is talking about, and you just pray that you don't start snoring or you're totally screwed. Thank goodness for lunch to get you chipper again, and because you're going to the gym after work, you figure you can afford a 'lil extra carbs. And maybe another coffee, just because, well, it's been *that* kind of day.

Now it's 3 p.m. and you're counting down the minutes until you can reunite with your pillow. Your soft, comfy, luxurious bamboo-threaded pillow. Yep, that's where you're headed straight after work. What? The gym? Dang. Not happening. You feel guilty for all of about 30 seconds as you contemplate the idea, but then you convince yourself that you are just too darn tired. So you figure you'll just skip dinner in lieu of working out, get a good night's sleep, and will for sure get up early the next morning and hit the gym when you are more energized. And the vicious cycle continues. The only exercise you get is lugging that gym bag around with you every day with the intention of doing some kind of physical activity. But you just don't... have... the energy. Sound familiar?

Food, literally, is your fuel. It's what drives you, motivates you and gives you that extra pep in your step. It can help you wake up feeling all bright-eyed and bushy-tailed, even before your alarm goes off! Imagine that. But, as they say, if you put crapola in you get crapola out. The quality of your energy, vibrancy and *life* is a direct reflection of what you put in your chomper and assimilate. Those refined carbs, sugar fixes and caffeine-induced energy drinks only set you up to fail. They might jack you up temporarily, but will have you crashing before you even start whatever it was you needed the energy to do. They don't fix the core problem. And about that skipping meals business... also fail.

Now, you might already be eating well and working out, but still find you're not on your A-game. Here are some key nutrients that will have you putting the Energizer bunny up for some stiff competition.

Tyrosine
Tyrosine is a non-essential amino acid, meaning your body produces it on its own (via phenylalanine, another amino acid). However, it can also be obtained directly through diet. The reason why this amino acid is so fab is because it's a precursor to the neurotransmitter dopamine, which is responsible for motivation and drive. It's what gives us that "get up and go" feeling. You know, that one we're typically lacking when we'd rather stay in bed all day? (Unless of course you're staying in bed for other reasons also related to dopamine — see page 39, wink, wink.) Studies show that supplementing with tyrosine improves mental and physical endurance, especially during times of stress.

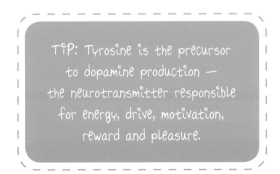

TIP: Tyrosine is the precursor to dopamine production — the neurotransmitter responsible for energy, drive, motivation, reward and pleasure.

Iron

Iron deficiency is a significant cause of fatigue, low energy and anemia, especially in women. Without enough iron, your body can't produce enough hemoglobin, which is a type of protein in red blood cells that enables them to carry oxygen throughout your body, giving it energy. The more oxygen getting to your cells, the more energetic and vibrant you'll be!

Heme iron (animal products)

Heme iron is derived from hemoglobin and is the most absorbable form of iron. It comes from animal sources such as clams, red meat, pork, chicken and fish.

Non-heme iron (plant-based foods, dairy and eggs)

The majority of dietary iron comes from non-heme sources. Unfortunately, it's not absorbed as well as heme iron. However, no need to fret — pairing up these foods with vitamin C helps to increase absorption. For example, adding lemon juice (source of vitamin C) to chickpeas (source of iron) or eating hummus with raw red peppers (excellent source of vitamin C) will increase the absorption of iron.

> Plant-based sources of iron: Lentils, Quinoa, Beans, Blackstrap Molasses, Amaranth, Spinach, Oatmeal, Raisins.

Try the following combos to maximize iron absorption:

Iron		Vitamin C
Hummus		Red peppers
Lentils		Parsley and lemon
Quinoa	*with*	Blackcurrants
Oatmeal		Strawberries
Spinach		Garlic

Factors that decrease iron absorption

Calcium, tannins (found in wine and tea) and phytates (found in legumes and whole grains) decrease iron absorption, so it's best to avoid eating these foods at the same time as iron-rich foods.

B-vitamins

B-vitamins are coined as the "energy" vitamins and are essential for mental and physical health and vitality — they're a pick-me-up for both mind and body! They help convert carbs, proteins and fats into usable energy. While all B-vitamins are essential and work synergistically together, B12 is probably the most important when it comes to boosting energy levels. B12, also known as cobalamine, is also required for the production of red blood cells, helps your body use iron, supports the immune system, and is used in the treatment and prevention of many diseases and mental health disorders. Unfortunately, getting enough B12 is one area where most people fall short.

> TIP: Be sure to consume calcium and iron at DIFFERENT times of the day to ensure maximum absorption of each.

Many North Americans are B12-deficient. Although vitamin B12 is difficult to obtain from plant-based sources, that doesn't let omnivores get off scot-free! It all depends on the state of your intestinal health, your stomach's ability to produce intrinsic factor, and re-absorption. B12 is a bacterial-synthesizing vitamin and is made solely out of microorganisms. Your body actually manufactures B12 through its own good bacteria, and much of it can be stored in the liver. As a result, most B12 deficiencies are due to the body's inability to perform in these key areas:

- The stomach needs to produce enough intrinsic factor, which is a protein released by the stomach lining that then latches onto B12 to help your body to absorb it.
- The stomach must produce enough hydrochloric acid (HCl) to pull out the B12 from your food (see Chapter 11 for more info on HCl), so if you have digestive issues, this may be a problem.
- B12 is excreted from the bile and reabsorbed. Deficiently could result from lack of re-absorption.

Although algaes are rich in B12, avoid relying on them as your sole source as absorption and bioavailability may be less than optimal. Your best bet is to use a high-quality supplement to meet your daily requirements

TOP ENERGY-BOOSTING FOODS

Chlorella
Chlorella is a green, single-celled, freshwater-grown algae and is one of the highest sources of chlorophyll in the *world*. It also boasts an amazing concentration of protein, vitamins, minerals and those precious trace-minerals for optimal health. Its rich chlorophyll content increases the number of red blood cells in your body, which help deliver oxygen to your cells. The more oxygen to

your cells, the more nutrients will be absorbed and the more *energy* you will have. Chlorophyll also boosts immune function, reduces inflammation and promotes alkalinity. The more alkaline your body, the healthier and more vibrant you will look and feel.

An amazing phenomenon of chlorella is the Chlorella Growth Factor (CGF), which means that this little microscopic alga spreads faster than a run in your tights. Seriously. It literally quadruples itself every 20 to 24 hours, making it the fastest-growing plant in the world! And now why would you want to ingest that? This jacked-up superfood increases tissue-building and repair (helping you look and feel fab), multiplies the 'good' active bacterial culture in your intestines (improving digestion and assimilation of nutrients and energy) and supercharges white blood cell activity. All of this boosts your immune system, health and vitality. Feeling pumped already? Yep. Thought so.

But wait. There's more.

Chlorella contains one of the highest food sources of RNA. RNA is a nucleic acid similar to DNA and an essential component of all life forms. It regulates gene expression, synthesizes proteins and helps DNA copy and express genetic material. Dr. Benjamin S. Frank pioneered the research behind RNA therapy. His work concluded that supplementing with foods rich in RNA increases energy and endurance, improves oxygen utilization, boosts the immune system, detoxifies and repairs cell damage and counteracts the effects of aging. He suggested that nucleic acids significantly increase cellular energy and rejuvenation. The greatest benefits are seen with those who are ill, have compromised immune systems or have undergone chemotherapy. The CGF is made up of these nucleic acids (RNA/DNA) in addition to proteins, peptides, polysaccharides, beta glucans, sulfur and manganese, which are found in the nucleus of the cell. This forms the core of chlorella's medicinal properties. Therefore, the higher the CGF, the better it is.

TIP: Chlorella contains up to five times more chlorophyll than wheat grass, up to 10 times more than spirulina, up to 12 times more than barley, and up to 50 times more than alfalfa (depending on species and grade).

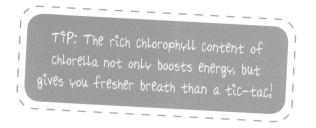

But we can't stop there! Chlorella is also rich in protein. At 60 per cent, chlorella has 12 times more digestible protein than beef! This helps balance blood sugar levels and wards off hunger and carb/sugar cravings. Protein also provides sustainable energy so you don't experience those crazy spikes and dips that have you raiding the vending machine mid-afternoon.

Chlorella is high in iodine, which is critical for healthy thyroid function. Your thyroid absorbs iodine from your blood in order to manufacture and distribute hormones throughout your body. If your blood is deficient in iodine, your thyroid won't be able to function properly. A sluggish thyroid causes your metabolism to slow down considerably, making you feel fatigued and, unfortunately, fat. Low thyroid levels can result in increased weight-gain and health risks.

See what I mean? Chlorella rocks. It's rich in energy-boosting and stress-busting B-vitamins, especially B1, B2 and B6, in addition to antioxidant-rich vitamins A, C and E. Chlorella has strong detoxification properties and helps remove heavy metals, pesticides and other toxins from the body (including alcohol!). FYI — it makes a great hangover remedy. Pop back some chlorella tabs before and after a night of drinking and it'll help cleanse alcohol from your liver. Plus, the high protein content will balance out your blood sugar levels, if you just so happened to indulge.

DID YOU KNOW?
Taking chlorella before and after a night of drinking helps your liver detox alcohol and can help with hangover symptoms. A Japanese study showed it can reduce the incidence of hangovers by 96 per cent!

HOW TO USE: To really boost energy, swap out your morning java for chlorella. It will have you feeling so energized you'll be fist-pumping all the way to work. 'Kay, maybe not exactly, but over time, you will notice a *huge* difference in energy levels. For optimal health, two to three grams per day is suggested. It can be taken any time of the day with or without food; however, it's best to take it in the morning, so it can boost your energy levels all day long. Make sure to get chlorella that's had the cell wall broken or cracked to ensure absorption and digestibility. Because of its detox properties, you may initially experience some symptoms such as nausea, acne or flu-like feelings if your system is heavily polluted. You can get it in tablet form (which is the easiest, most convenient and palatable form), or you can get it in powder form and add it to smoothies or juices.

Another way to get chlorella as well as a whole host of other nutritional goodness like protein, fibre, greens and omega-3 is in Vega Whole Food Health Optimizer. The Vega line was created by a friend of mine, Brendan Brazier, who is a professional vegan triathlete and best-selling author on performance nutrition. I add a bit of the smoothie powder to my breakfast smoothie regularly. And if you're still thinking about how chlorella can be used as a hangover remedy, check out my recipe which includes Vega on page 133.

> TIP: A diet rich in chlorophyll is like giving your blood an instant transfusion of goodness! It enhances the ability of red blood cells to carry oxygen, strengthens our immune system and fends off disease.

Sunflower sprouts
Sunflower sprouts are "micro-greens" sprouted from the sunflower seed and harvested in the beginning stages of their growth. This is when the plants are the most nutrient-dense, bio-available and enzyme-rich. These crisp, fresh-tasting sprouts are rich in protein, vitamins (including B and D), enzymes and phytonutrients, which help protect against disease.

When sprouting, the nutritional profile of sunflower sprouts can increase anywhere from 100 to 600 per cent, making sprouts superior to any other leafy (macro) green. They are higher in chlorophyll than any macro green, increasing the number of red blood cells that deliver oxygen to your cells. They also have amazing detoxification properties. These sprouts are extremely alkalizing, with several healing properties. Benefits include blood purification, cancer prevention, improved circulation and strengthened immune system. Eat these raw and as close to harvest as possible for maximum nutritional benefit!

Sunflower sprouts are one of the most enzyme-rich foods around. Enzymes are the catalysts of all life. They spark the electrical conduit for every chemical reaction that occurs in our body. They help repair skin, recover from illnesses, heal wounds and digest food. We are born with a full bank of enzymes. However, over time, stresses from our environment, nutritionally-void food and negative thoughts deplete the number of enzymes, and the aging process and cellular degradation occurs. This is why eating foods rich in enzymes is so important — they add to our "bank." And raw, plant-based foods are the only natural source.

HOW TO USE: Do not cook these! It's important to eat them raw, as cooking will destroy the precious nutrients and enzymes that make these sprouts so powerful. Sunflower sprouts make a great base or addition to a salad. They can be added to sandwiches and wraps, topped on soups or rolled into sushi rolls. Juicing sunflower sprouts provides great detoxification as well as blood- and liver-cleansing benefits. Juice or blend with cucumber, apple, lemon and ginger for a refreshing and cleansing cocktail!

> TiP: Soak all seeds, grains and legumes eight to 12 hours before consuming or cooking. This process activates enzymes and pre-digests macronutrients (carbs, proteins and fats), allowing your body to more easily assimilate the nutrients.

Sea veggies
Sea veggies are just that — veggies grown in the sea! Some varieties include arame, nori, kelp, wakame and dulse. Just like land-grown veggies, sea veggies are uber-high in vitamins, minerals and phytonutrients. However, they are also laced with beneficial trace minerals difficult to get from any other food source. Your body needs minerals to create energy-producing reactions in your cells, and sea veggies are loaded with them! They also are some of the highest plant-based sources of iron, and because they are also rich in vitamin C, the bioavailability of the iron is increased.

Sea veggies are also rich in the amino acid tyrosine, which is a precursor to dopamine production. Dopamine is the neurotransmitter that gives us that energy to get up and go! It's what stimulates drive and motivation. It's what lights the fire under your butt to get moving when you're feeling lazy. It's known to 'rev-up' the brain, which can help you feel more alert and focused. Who couldn't benefit from that?

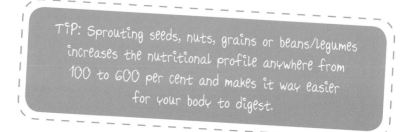

TIP: Sprouting seeds, nuts, grains or beans/legumes increases the nutritional profile anywhere from 100 to 600 per cent and makes it way easier for your body to digest.

Sea veggies also have exceptionally high iodine content. Iodine is essential for thyroid function. Your thyroid must absorb sufficient amounts of iodine from your blood in order to manufacture and distribute hormones throughout your body. If the thyroid is sluggish and not functioning optimally, your metabolism slows, and an onset of fatigue and lethargy kicks in — which means you feel lazy, and maybe even fat. By incorporating sea veggies into your diet, especially kelp, which has the highest iodine content, you can ensure you'll feel fab!

HOW TO USE: Sea veggies typically come dried and can be rehydrated in water for about five minutes. Arame and wakame are great additions to salads or soups, or sprinkled on top of steamed veggies. They also make a great salad on their own, drizzled with some sesame oil. They add a nice saltiness to dishes. Nori is typically used to roll up veggies or maki rolls and makes a great snack on its own. Kelp and dulse also come in granules, and although they look like pepper, they taste like salt! They make a great salt substitute — just sprinkle the granules on top of your food for a great mineral boost. My favourite way to eat dulse is in a DLT — dulse, lettuce and tomato sandwich, with a little avocado for good measure!

The hierarchy of greens based on nutrient density and chlorophyll levels:

Good	Better	Best	Bestest!
Macro Greens	Micro Greens	Sea Veggies	Algaes
Dark leafy greens: *Kale* *Spinach* *Collards* *Mustards* *greens, etc.*	Sprouts: *Sunflower* *sprouts* *Pea sprouts* *Buckwheat* *sprouts* *Broccoli sprouts* *Sprouted* *legumes*	Kelp Dulse Nori Wakame Arame Hijiki	Chlorella Spirulina AFA

Clams

Here's another nutrient-rich sea creature. Although not a plant, clams boast the highest concentration of heme iron, which is the most bioavailable form of iron.

Iron deficiency is a significant cause of fatigue, low energy and anemia, especially in women. Without enough iron, your body can't produce enough hemoglobin, which means your red blood cells can't carry enough oxygen to your body. And oxygen equals energy! At roughly 23 milligrams of iron per three-ounce serving, clams are one of the highest food sources of this energy-boosting nutrient.

Clams are also an excellent source of vitamin B12 and can give you over seven times the recommended daily amount! B12 is essential to boosting energy levels and mental concentration, and aids in the absorption of iron and the production of red blood cells. The iron-B12 combo of clams is a surefire way to boost energy.

Added bonus! Clams are also rich in protein, helping balance blood sugar levels and provide sustainable energy to last throughout the day!

HOW TO USE: Purchase live, fresh clams that are 'clammed' tightly shut! Once they've been cooked, discard the clams that don't open, as they were dead prior to cooking. You can add them to your favourite pasta dish, or they taste delish on their own in a tomato or herbed white wine sauce.

Water
The most common cause of fatigue is dehydration! If there is not enough fluid in your body, blood volume can drop. As a result, your body (and heart) must work harder in order to supply you cells with oxygen and nutrients. Poor hydration results in mental fogginess, poor short-term memory, dizziness and fatigue. How much should you drink every day? A good rule of thumb is to drink half your body weight (lbs) in ounces. So if you weigh 130 lbs, you need 65 ounces of water a day — just over eight cups. If you want more energy in your day, drink up!

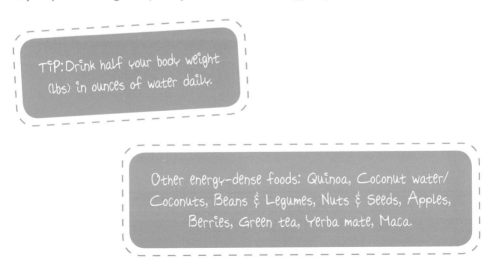

TIP: Drink half your body weight (lbs) in ounces of water daily.

Other energy-dense foods: Quinoa, Coconut water/ Coconuts, Beans & Legumes, Nuts & Seeds, Apples, Berries, Green tea, Yerba mate, Maca.

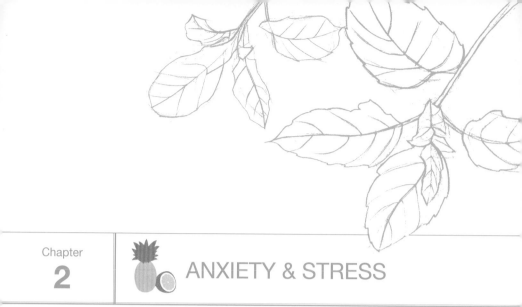

ANXIETY & STRESS

Whether you are rushing to get out of the house in the morning, are about to give a huge presentation, are worried about finances, had too many martinis, are wondering why he didn't call, are wondering why he didn't call while drinking too many martinis, sprained an ankle, broke a heel, feel overwhelmed with life, lost your job, started a new job, are trying to balance a career, children and a husband, or are just pulling your hair out trying to squeeze into a pair of jeans that you *swear* fit you just last week, you've been met with stress.

All types of stress, whether it is actual stress or something we just make up in our heads, cause a physiological response in our body. At the onset of stress, your brain triggers your adrenal glands, which sit on top of your kidneys, causing them to release the stress hormones adrenaline and cortisol. Adrenaline speeds up heart rate, increases blood pressure and boosts energy. Cortisol, which is the primary stress hormone, shifts energy away from the digestive and immune systems to prepare for an "alarmed" state and increases blood sugar levels and the brain's uptake of glucose.

Some stress is great. For example, if you're about to run a half marathon, those stress hormones pumping through your body might just give you the edge to run that much faster and stronger. It's the "fight or flight" response that revs up your body and makes it work hard. However, the key here is that it's finite. The race eventually ends and, in the process, you burn off all the elevated sugar and fat that were released as a response to stress through physical exertion. Your blood pressure drops, your heart rate slows and your body returns back to your normal state.

Where the problem lies is when there is ongoing, chronic stress — when there is no finish line, when one worry or stress is followed by another, and it just seems like it never ends. Day-to-day demands, worry, tension and poor lifestyle habits cause your adrenals to fire constantly, and cortisol levels are released in excess.

Here are some of the chronic effects of excess cortisol:
- Leads to weight-gain (especially belly fat!), obesity and inability to burn fat
- Interferes with the neurotransmitter serotonin, which can lead to clinical depression, anxiety disorders and insomnia
- Can cause mental clutter, poor concentration and impaired memory function
- Breaks down collagen and speeds up the aging process
- Increases blood pressure, blood clotting and cholesterol levels
- Suppresses the immune system and the function of pathogen-fighting T-cells
- Increases the risk of heart attack, stroke and kidney disease
- Promotes insulin resistance, which leads to additional belly fat
- Increases levels of estrogen, which also leads to weight-gain and mood swings
- Increases cravings

Basically, in time, it'll make you fat. And the end result: more stress.

Why do we crave certain foods when we're stressed? Take a look at what our cravings are really telling us:

Fats	Bad saturated and trans fats can numb the receptors in the brain that regulate emotional responses.
Carbs & Sugars	Carbohydrates help release serotonin, a neurotransmitter in our brain that makes us feel happy and relaxed. However, refined carbs and sugars cause blood sugar imbalances and lead to greater feelings of stress, anxiety and depression.
Salt	Stress depletes our body of precious minerals and throws off our sodium/potassium balance. Cortisol is also a natural diuretic, which can lead to dehydration, which can lead to salt cravings.
Chocolate	Chocolate releases endorphins, which alleviate pain, and may contain magnesium (if it's raw or extremely dark chocolate), which helps alleviate tension.

What you eat absolutely makes a difference to how your body deals with stress.

The problem is that when we're stressed and reach for the *wrong* types of food — foods that are nutritionally void and high in refined carbs, sugar, fats or caffeine — it further exacerbates our stress. These foods actually *cause* stress.

They worsen the symptoms and issues at hand. Caffeine and sugar stimulate the nervous system, increasing agitation and nervousness. High fat foods are difficult for your body to break down and digest, while foods that are just flat out nutritionally-void cause your body added stress, as they don't supply it with the precious nutrients it needs to function optimally.

Happy Hour

What about alcohol? A few glasses of wine are sure to take the edge off after a crazy day... right? Actually, it can. Alcohol increases the production of GABA, the neurotransmitter responsible for feelings of calm and relaxation. GABA is what squashes nervousness in social situations after a few drinks. It gets rid of hang-ups you initially had about that annoying dude who was hitting on you earlier on in the night, and lets down your guard, making you believe there is absolutely nothing wrong with drunk dialing at 3 a.m. It alleviates nervousness and tension and keeps you from being uptight. Perfect remedy for a first date or dinner with the in-laws, right? Maybe not so much.

The GABA kick via alcohol consumption is relatively short-lived. Once GABA plummets, it'll have you feeling *blah*. So chances are you'll reach for another drink and the vicious cycle will continue. It then goes on to interrupt your sleep and causes further stress, irritability and agitation. As for tranquillizers, such a Valium or Ativan, they are highly-addictive and can lead to further anxiety in the long run.

So for all you stress-cases and type-A personalities out there, here are some of the nutrients your body needs to chillax, au natural!

KEY STRESS-BUSTING NUTRIENTS

GABA

GABA is an amino acid and neurotransmitter that helps us chill. It's an "inhibitory" neurotransmitter (vs. "excitatory" like its dopamine counterpart). It promotes a feeling of calm and relaxation, and shuts off excess adrenaline.It helps to manage stress and improve mental focus — balancing out all those crazy thoughts. The best way to increase GABA production naturally and healthfully is through food. A precursor to GABA production is the amino acid glutamine. Hence, foods rich in glutamic acids (or glutamate) help increase GABA production.

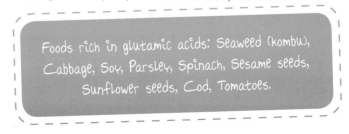

Foods rich in glutamic acids: Seaweed (kombu), Cabbage, Soy, Parsley, Spinach, Sesame seeds, Sunflower seeds, Cod, Tomatoes.

Adaptogens

Adaptogens are nutrients found in herbs that increase the body's ability to resist and adapt to stress. They can help alleviate anxiety, stress and trauma by restoring the body's natural balance and homeostasis.

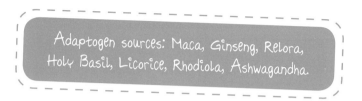

Adaptogen sources: Maca, Ginseng, Relora, Holy Basil, Licorice, Rhodiola, Ashwagandha.

Vitamin B6

B-vitamins are stress-busting. They are essential in the production of neurotransmitters (especially B6, B12, folic acid and niacin). Unfortunately, while B6 is the most important in terms of busting stress, it's also the first to be depleted in the presence of stress. A lack of B6 could lead to depression due to its inability to produce the feel-good neurotransmitter serotonin. And because B-vitamins are water-soluble, they don't hang around in your body very long — so it's essential we ingest them throughout the day.

Foods rich in Vitamin B6: Fatty fish (tuna), Red & green peppers, Cod, Hazelnuts, Cashew nuts, Potatoes, Spinach, Bananas, Turnip greens, Garlic, Cauliflower.

Vitamin C

Vitamin C is a powerful antioxidant. Not only does it help to protect against oxidative stress and free-radical damage as a result of physical stress, but vitamin C can also helps curb the large spikes in cortisol as a response to mental stress. In an animal study, rats that were not given vitamin C while undergoing stress experienced three times the level of cortisol than those that were supplemented with vitamin C.

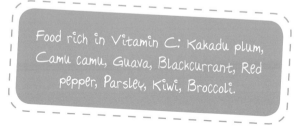

Food rich in Vitamin C: Kakadu plum, Camu camu, Guava, Blackcurrant, Red pepper, Parsley, Kiwi, Broccoli.

Calcium and magnesium

The minerals calcium and magnesium have calming effects on the body and nervous system. Deficiencies in these important minerals can aggravate anxiety and tension. Magnesium is one of the most common mineral deficiencies. It helps relax nerves and tense muscles, alleviate muscle-cramping and headaches, and can help you fall asleep. If supplementing, it's best to take before bed.

Food rich in calcium and magnesium:
Kale, Broccoli, Sesame seeds/ Tahini, Almonds, Maca, Sacha inchi seeds.

TIP: Omega-3 fatty acids also help alleviate anxiety and depression.

FOODS THAT HELP YOU CHILL

Holy Basil

Next time you're stuck in *holy traffic*, you might want to reach for some holy basil! Holy basil (also known as tulsi) is an herbal plant native to India but now cultivated all over the world. Oh, and by the way, it tastes nothing like the regular basil you're used to, so here's a word of advice — don't use it in pasta dishes! It's been used historically in Ayurvedic medicine to reduce fever, strengthen the immune system, calm nerves and act as an anti-inflammatory and antioxidant. However, more recent studies have shown that holy basil has the ability to lower cortisol and blood sugar levels — that is, help our bodies cope with stress!

Holy basil is an adaptogen, meaning it doesn't directly affect your mood, but it helps your body respond to stress, anxiety, trauma and depression by normalizing neurotransmitter levels in the brain. Research has shown that ursolic acid and the triterpenoic acids, both found in holy basil, effectively improve the body's response to stress, and reduce the amount of cortisol released during stress. Ursolic acid also has anti-cancer and anti-tumor properties — can't beat that! Additional compounds demonstrate anti-stress effects by normalizing blood sugar levels, cortisol levels and reducing the enlargement of the adrenal glands. In comparison to ginseng, another adaptogenic herb, holy basil exhibits greater anti-stress properties, with a higher margin of safety.

Researchers at the Dr. B.C. Roy Institute of Post Graduate Medical Education and Research in India screened 35 subjects with generalized anxiety disorder (GAD) in a clinical investigation. Each subject was given 500 milligrams of holy basil twice a day. After 60 days, it was observed that the severity of GAD-associated stress and depression was significantly reduced in the subjects.

Holy basil also contains various other therapeutic compounds, such as rosmarinic acid, which has anti-inflammatory properties and can help reduce inflammation of the adrenal glands. Holy basil also has strong antioxidant properties, which helps protect your body from the free-radical damage associated with stress. In addition, it also contains oleanolic acids, which have strong anti-tumor and anti-viral (including anti-HIV) properties.

HOW TO USE: Holy basil has a spicy, clove-like flavour and is not traditionally used in cooking (except in Thai cooking for hot stir-fries and curries). It's mainly used in North America as a supplement — typically as a soft gel containing standardized holy basil leaf extract in an oil base (look for supercritical extract). You can also find it as whole dried leaf capsules, in a tea form (tulsi tea) or as seed oil.

Raw Chocolate
Who doesn't feel good after eating chocolate? Chocolate is the number one craved food in the world, and a survey suggested that 50 per cent of women would rather eat chocolate than have sex! Chocolate releases the same feel-good endorphins that suppress pain and stress, and gives the same euphoric feeling you get from having sex or going for a run. But it's the raw chocolate (aka cacao) where all the good stuff is stored — so step away from the vending machines! Raw chocolate is rich in antioxidants, minerals and stress-alleviating compounds, giving you a guilt-free boost.

Cacao contains a compound called phenylethylamine (PEA), which promotes a happy, elated feeling and alleviates stress and depression. They call it the "love molecule," as it raises your pulse and gives you that same feeling you get while falling in love. In addition, pure, raw chocolate is also one of the highest sources of magnesium. Magnesium is essential in reducing muscle-tension, calming the nerves and promoting relaxation. Chocolate also contains a neurotransmitter known as anandamide that has the ability to alter dopamine levels in the brain, causing a sense of peace and relaxation. And it gets even better — cacao is rich in B-vitamins, which help the body cope with stress. So if you're looking to de-stress and relax, a piece of raw chocolate should do the trick!

Stress can have a profound negative impact on your heart, including elevated blood pressure and increased risk of heart attack. But cacao can help counter the negative effects of stress on heart health. A team of researchers at the University of Adelaide in Australia found that for those with high blood pressure, the flavonols found in chocolate reduced blood pressure to a similar degree as 30 minutes of physical activity! This could reduce the risk of a cardiovascular event by 20 per cent over five years.

Cacao also has an exceptionally high ORAC value, which is the measurement of antioxidant activity. It trumps blueberries and pomegranates in levels of antioxidants, making it an amazingly delicious way to prevent against oxidative stress, free-radical damage and disease.

HOW TO USE: Raw cacao can be a bit bitter, especially if you're used to "fake" chocolate laced in sugar, with most of the *actual* chocolate removed. But no need to fret — you can have your chocolate and eat it too, in a way that's divinely decadent and delish. Check out some of my recipes in the back of the book! You can add cacao nibs or powder to breakfast cereals, smoothies, homemade granola, tossed into trail mix, made into a rich hot cocoa or added to your favourite desserts. Alternatively you can find some heavenly raw chocolate bars or bars with high cocoa content on the market.

> TIP: Cocoa powder is when fat is removed from the cacao bean and ground into a powder. Cocoa butter is solely the fat from the cacao bean. White chocolate is NOT really chocolate! It's just the fat (cocoa butter) mixed with sugar, amongst other stuff!

Passionflower
I know what you're thinking — shouldn't *passion*flower be in the chapter on sex? Despite its name, passionflower is primarily known as a calming herb. It grows in many parts of the world, but is native to North, Central and South America. Passionflower has been used for years to treat anxiety, stress, insomnia and nervousness. The second half of its name is also misleading! The actual medicinal benefits are found in the stem and root of the plant, not in the flower itself. It is used as an herbal remedy in a tea form or as a liquid extract or capsule.

Passionflower has mild sedative and tranquilizing effects that can calm nerves and reduce anxiety, and is without addictive properties. A study in the *Journal of Clinical Pharmacy and Therapeutics* indicated that passionflower was just as effective as the prescription medication Oxazepam in the treatment of generalized anxiety disorder (GAD), and did not have any of the side effects such as impaired job performance. Out of the 36 subjects with GAD, half were given 45 drops of passionflower extract per day, and the other half were given 30 milligrams of Oxazepam per day. After the four-week trial, there was no significant difference between the two groups. The study also determined that passionflower also increases the levels of the neurotransmitter GABA that helps with calm and relaxation.

Chrysin, which is a flavonoid compound found in passionflower, has anti-anxiety effects. Chrysin is also a powerful antioxidant and anti-inflammatory that helps to protect against disease and the aging process. In particular, it has the ability to inhibit COX-2 and 5-lipoxygenase enzymes, which play a role in inflammation and pain, as well as Alzheimer's disease, respectively. In addition, this flavonoid also has libido-boosting properties, as it can inhibit the conversion of testosterone to estrogen. So maybe there's some passion in this flower after all! Researchers in India reported that when Chrysin was combined with benzoflavone moiety (BZF) it increased the sexual function of aging rats. Hmm. Perhaps the anti-anxiety effects knocked out performance anxiety?

HOW TO USE: Passionflower can be enjoyed as a relaxing tea or taken in liquid or capsule form. Passionflower works synergistically with valerian and lemon balm, and the three are often combined to treat insomnia. For adults, 100 to 250 milligrams a day is generally recommended to promote relaxation and alleviate symptoms of nervousness, tension or anxiety. From 100 to 200 milligrams per day can also help reduce hyperactivity in kids.

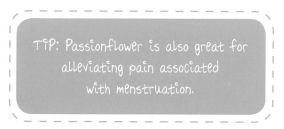

TIP: Passionflower is also great for alleviating pain associated with menstruation.

Sweet potato

When you're totally maxed out and in search for some good comfort food to feed your soul, look no further than the sweet and starchy sweet potato. This delish root veg is jam-packed with stress-busting nutrients, including vitamin B6, vitamin C, antioxidant beta-carotene and calcium.

Carbohydrates get a bad rap, but they can, in fact, help chill you out. Studies show that carbs can reduce stress levels, improve mental performance and can help mitigate stress-induced depression. They increase serotonin levels in the brain, our feel-good neurotransmitter, and promote a feeling of calmness. This is why we tend to reach for carbs when we're feeling overwhelmed, because they physiologically make us feel better. However, the issue lies in the type of carbs consumed. Simple, refined carbs such as refined breads, sugars and white pasta may make us feel better temporarily, but the effects are extremely short-lived. Then they leave us feeling bloated, fat, depressed and even more stressed, so we continue to eat more simple carbs, and the vicious cycle continues.

On the other hand, complex carbohydrates such as sweet potatoes, quinoa and oats are slow-releasing carbs that keep you more satiated and feeling less anxious for longer periods of time. When we're stressed, our cortisol levels are elevated and our blood glucose levels increase, which means ongoing stress can totally muck up blood sugar levels. But sweet potatoes actually help balance blood sugar levels, making them a great stress antidote. They increase blood levels of a hormone called adiponectin, which regulates the metabolism of insulin; contain phytic acids, which lower blood glucose levels; and also contain caiapo (found in white sweet potatoes), which Austrian researchers indicate improves metabolic control by lowering insulin resistance in type II diabetics. So, energy levels will be balanced, cravings controlled and anxiety levels managed! Sweet!

Sweet potatoes are a rich source of B-vitamins, especially B5 and B6, which support and calm the nervous system and play a key role in the production of neurotransmitters. They are also rich in antioxidant vitamins A (beta carotene) and C, which are essential for protecting the body from the free-radical damage caused by stress. Vitamin C also keeps your immune system in check, which tends to suffer during stressful times. Because vitamin C and the B-vitamins are water-soluble, they don't last very long in your body and need to be replenished frequently, especially during times of stress. Sweet potatoes, especially the purple varieties, are also high in anthocyanins — a powerful antioxidant that combats the effects of stress, aging and cognitive decline. They also contain calcium and magnesium, two important minerals for calming and relaxing muscles and nerves.

TiP: Fats increase the absorption of beta-carotene, so eat sweet potatoes with a little drizzle of extra virgin olive oil, hemp seed oil, or even coconut butter... YUM!

TiP: Cooking sweet potatoes lowers their glycemic index — which is a good thing, because they taste WAY better that way!

Almonds
Misery loves company. If you feel like you're going nuts, you might as well start adding them to your diet! These bite-size gems are the perfect snack food for those times you feel like crawling under a rock. Almonds are fantastic stress

relievers; they're packed with loads of essential vitamins, minerals and nutrients that support mental health and help you achieve a calm, cool mind. Almonds contain some of the most important mood-enhancing nutrients, including vitamin B2 (riboflavin), magnesium, vitamin E and zinc.

Almonds are a great source of many B-vitamins, which are essential for smooth nervous system function. Almonds are especially high in vitamin B2, which helps produce anti-stress hormones, including serotonin — our all-time "happy" neurotransmitter. Almonds also have tons of magnesium. High levels of magnesium support a relaxed mind and body and promote nervous system health. Magnesium also activates many enzymes required for energy production in the body, which is key when stress is high and immune function is low. As B-vitamins and magnesium are both involved in the production of serotonin, they can further help regulate mood and relieve stress.

Almonds also contain high levels of zinc, which is crucial for the immune system, an area that often takes a beating when you're stressed. For this reason, zinc has been shown to fight the negative effects of stress and anxiety. Vitamin E, also found in almonds, is an antioxidant that destroys free radicals related to stress. Because vitamin E reduces oxidative stress, that translates to reduced stress in the body. Almonds also contain omega-3 fatty acids, which are essential for proper brain function and lower levels of the stress hormone cortisol, reducing feelings of stress and anxiety in the body and mind.

HOW TO USE: With all these positive health effects, it is easy to want to overload on these highly nutritious goodies, but it's important to keep in mind that these little guys are still high in calories and fat (even if it's the good kind). As with everything, they should be consumed in moderation. A couple of tablespoons two or three times a week is more than enough to get that desired calming effect. Be sure to each almonds raw, not roasted, as roasting depletes many of the nutritional benefits.

The skin of almonds contains enzyme inhibitors that keep almonds in a dormant state. Since almonds are a living food, these enzyme inhibitors are what prevent them from growing just by sitting on your counters. But they can also make it difficult for them to be broken down in your body. This is why it is best to soak almonds in water for eight to 12 hours before eating. The enzyme inhibitors are released during the soaking process and the nut begins to germinate. Many of the fats are released (making it a slightly lower-calorie nut!), and the macronutrients (proteins and fats) are broken down into a pre-digestible form, making it easier to digest and assimilate the nutrients. Once they are done soaking, give them a good rinse and munch away! If you miss the crunch (and chances are if you are stressed you LOVE the crunch), just lightly toast them at a super-low temperature to maintain the nutritional benefits.

Relora

Introduced as a natural health product in the last decade, the herbs that make up Relora have been used traditionally for centuries. Relora is an entirely natural dietary supplement that helps combat the effects of stress on the body. Not only does this wonder supplement help alleviate stress, it also counteracts stress-related eating, promotes healthy weight loss and has amazing anti-aging benefits, which gives you a few less things to be stressed about!

Relora is a combination of two active herbal plant extracts commonly used in traditional Chinese medicine — magnolia officinalis and phellodendron amurense. Both those in the field of alternative medicine and in the medical community have praised it for its efficacy. Relora works by quieting the functioning of the endocrine organs (like the adrenal and pituitary glands), lessening the effect stress has on the body. The active ingredients in Relora bind to receptor target sites in the central nervous system that are associated with stress and anxiety. Studies have shown much success with diet and stress levels while supplementing with Relora. Not only does it moderate hormone levels, but also seems to limit an individual's *perceived* level of stress. As a dietary aid, Relora inhibits the production of cortisol, an excess of which can prevent weight loss. And although it is non-drowsy in nature, it has also proven effective for those suffering from stress-related insomnia.

If the stress-busting, weight-loss benefits weren't enough to get you running for some Relora, it also has amazing anti-aging benefits! Relora naturally increases DHEA, which is our body's anti-aging, anti-stress hormone. It's like our rock star hormone, and with it kicking full throttle in our bodies, it helps reduce body fat, increases lean muscle and keeps us youthful! Studies show that the benefits of using Relora can be seen in as quickly as two weeks!

HOW TO USE: Relora is non-habit forming and can be taken by anyone trying to relieve stress or lose weight in a healthy way. However, it should be used in conjunction with an exercise plan and a fresh, whole food diet for best results. If you're taking Relora for stress, anxiety or other mood disorders, it should be taken as part of a complete wellness plan. It's also best to consume on an empty stomach and prior to going to bed.

	Here are some more key stress-busting tips:
1	Add real, nutrient-dense, stress-busting foods to your diet.
2	Exercise, practice yoga, meditate.
3	Hang out with the girls! Yep — some good quality bonding time with your fave gal pals is one of the most powerful ways to reduce stress and boost your health! Just as good as, if not better than, exercise!
4	Get some good shut-eye. Sleep helps regulate cortisol levels.
5	Journal. Get all that crap out of your head (and body) and onto paper.
6	Think happy thoughts. Most of the stress in our life is perceived stress — things we create in our head. Change the way you look at and think about things. Find a new perspective. Always think in the positive. Shiny, happy thoughts!
7	Take a deeeep breath and…
8	LAUGH OUT LOUD!

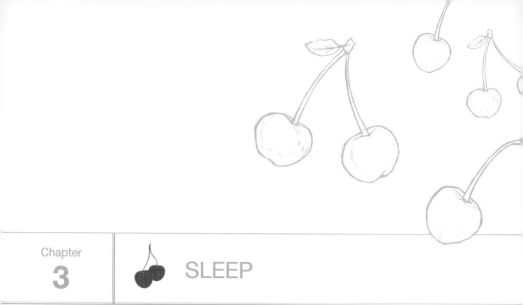

SLEEP

Count sheep? Who the heck has time for that when there are way more important things to think about, like whether or not you *really* have to return that hot new pair of Louboutins in order to make your rent payment? Or how to face your boss tomorrow knowing you didn't hit your deadline on time, but still need to leave work early to take your kid to soccer practice. Regardless of what's keeping you up at night — relationships, work stress, financial matters, family — getting enough zzz's is totally underrated.

What promotes sleepiness: understanding melatonin

Tic-tock people, tic-tock. Whether we like it or not, our bodies operate on an internal clock. Not the "Holy crap, I'm getting old!" clock, but the circadian clock, and it's constantly ticking. Circadian rhythms tell our body when it's time to sleep and when it's time to wake. And unfortunately there is no snooze button. It's totally influenced by our environment. When night falls, darkness triggers the production of melatonin. Melatonin, secreted by the pineal gland in the brain, is a hormone and antioxidant responsible for sleep. The darker it becomes, the more melatonin is secreted; as it becomes lighter, melatonin decreases. But since we're living in the age of florescent lights, city lights, computer screens and PVR, we totally mess up our body's innate ability to sleep soundly. So, what's a girl got to do to get some good shut-eye?

1	**Sleep in complete darkness.** Yes, that means no sleeping with your Blackberry or television. Even the light from your alarm clock can prevent you from getting your beauty sleep. The blue light that is emitted from your television, digital clocks and media devices interferes with melatonin production. If you do need an alarm clock, opt for one with red lights, as red has a more calming effect on the brain. Even better, invest in one that gradually wakes you up with light or soft sounds.
2	**Don't eat before bed.** Contrary to popular opinion, eating before bed will not lead to weight-gain, but it will disrupt your sleep. Laying down post-nosh will lead to indigestion, leaving you wrestling with your sheets.
3	**Avoid stimulating foods, such as caffeine or alcohol.** Even though we're convinced a glass (or four) of red wine will knock us out at night, its effects won't last very long and will keep us up most of the night.
4	**Cool down.** If room temperatures are too high (over 21 degrees Celsius), it may prevent you from getting your best sleep. Body temperature typically drops when you fall asleep, so a cooler room temperature is more aligned to your body's own innate sleep temperature.
5	**Sleep or have sex.** Those are the only two things you should be doing in your bed. Period.

Why you need your sleep

Need to lie on your bed just to squeeze into your skinny jeans? Get more shut-eye during the night and you'll be sliding into them like a pair of cashmere gloves. Women who sleep fewer than seven hours a night are likely to gain more weight than those who get seven-plus hours of sleep. If that's not enough reason to hit the hay, sleep deprivation also causes extreme stress on your body. Not only will it make you all moody and bitch-faced, it also affects your concentration, memory and reaction time, depletes your body of nutrients such as zinc, and pretty much sucks dry *all* vitamin C. Sleep deprivation can also elevate blood pressure and increase your risk of diabetes and cancer. Studies show that women who work shift work have higher incidences of breast cancer. Melatonin, which is produced during sleep, slows down estrogen levels. If we're not sleeping well, melatonin production is reduced and excess estrogen, which is linked to breast cancer, is kickin' full throttle. But it's not limited to just "the girls." Since melatonin is also an antioxidant, a decrease in production means less juice to give cancer-causing free-radical damage a kick in the ass. Research also shows that melatonin can stop the growth of cancer cells dead in their tracks for many cancers, including colorectal, prostate and liver; whereas a decrease in melatonin can rapidly accelerate tumor growth. Not cool.

It's when we're sound asleep that our body is the most efficient and working the hardest to heal and repair itself from the day's abuses. Cortisol levels are restored, cells are regenerated, human growth hormone (hGH) is secreted, fat is burned, and the liver detoxs — just to name a few. So the more hours you sacrifice of sleep, the more you're missing out on being your best self.

SLEEPY-TIME FOODS

Tart cherries

Our precious antioxidant/neurotransmitter melatonin is not only produced by our pineal gland, but can also be found in some plant-based foods in high concentrations — in particular, Montmorency tart cherries. Yes, these tart cherries (aka sour cherries) are the same ones found in your favourite cherry pie. The two main varieties of tart cherries are Montmorency cherries, which are bright red sour cherries, and Balaton cherries, which are darker in colour and have more of a sweet/ sour taste. Although all varieties of tart cherries contain the highest plant-based source of readily absorbable dietary melatonin, Montmorency cherries contain six times more than the Balaton variety. A study conducted by the University of Rochester Medical Center concluded that the consumption of tart cherry juice significantly reduced the severity of insomnia and reduced "wake periods" after sleep onset. Although it won't necessarily get you to sleep quicker, once you fall asleep, it'll keep you there, versus waking up and staying awake throughout the night.

In addition to all this sleep-enhancing goodness, these delish little morsels also contain a decent dose of anthocyanins, which can reduce oxidative stress, inhibit the growth of cancer cells and help prevent diseases such as atherosclerosis, diabetes and Alzheimer's disease. And for all you athletic types, research also suggests that tart cherry juice makes a phenomenal sports recovery drink. The antioxidant, anti-inflammatory properties help reduce muscle damage, inflammation, pain, and oxidative stress associated with endurance training. Tart cherry juice also helps speed up the recovery of muscle function. In a study published in the *Journal of the International Society of Sports Nutrition*, researchers at Oregon Health and Science University's Department of Medicine suggested that ingesting tart cherry juice for seven days prior to and during a strenuous running event can minimize post-run muscle pain. Less pain, better sleep and better health all around!

HOW TO USE: Tart cherries can be consumed as a concentrated juice, in supplement powder form or by just eating the cherries on their own! For maximum sleep benefit, drinking one or two eight-ounce glasses of the juice daily or eating approximately 20 to 25 whole cherries should do the trick. When eating the cherries whole, please don't go for the can of pie filling! Those cherries have been cooked to death, are completely devoid of any nutritional benefit and are laced with fat-causing sugar. Trust me — a week of that and you won't be happy, just fat and probably sleep-deprived. But no need to fret — be sure to check out my guilt-free, absolutely scrumptious Choco Cherry Smoothie recipe on page 135! You can find them whole, frozen or dried at most major health food stores.

Valerian root

Valerian is a perennial plant native to Europe and Asia, but which now grows in North America. It's known for its sedative properties and is used in the treatment of insomnia and anxiety. Who needs to count sheep? Valerian's sedative effects speed up the initial falling asleep process. While it may not necessarily improve the quality of sleep like tart cherries do, it makes the process of getting there a little less painful.

There are a variety of components found in valerian root that work together to make it happen. GABA, which is our relaxing neurotransmitter, is typically present in valerian root extract. However, it's not necessarily the GABA in the extract that causes the sedation, as it's difficult for GABA to cross the blood-brain barrier. Instead, valerian increases the release of GABA from the brain's nerve endings and prevents the re-absorption of GABA into the synaptic cleft. Studies show that the efficacy of valerian root has a cumulative effect and happens over time with daily use, versus using it as a one-shot sleeping aide. In addition, the fact that it helps to reduce anxiety contributes to the fact that it helps induce sleep. You know those nights when you're bone-tired and yet you lie awake for hours while your mind goes 'round and 'round in circles about all the stuff that's stressing you out? The less stressed and anxious we are, especially at bedtime, the quicker we'll fall asleep, and valerian is a great combo stress-buster and sleep-inducer.

HOW TO USE: Valerian can be consumed as a tea or herbal tincture, in which the oil is extracted from the dried root. Research shows that approximately 600 to 1,000 milligrams of the extract should be consumed for it to work effectively. If greater amounts are taken, some report a feeling of drowsiness in the morning — not what we're going for here! Just add some drops of valerian extract to passionflower or chamomile tea, which also has calming effects, for a soothing bedtime tea. Keep in mind that valerian root extract smells and tastes, well, pretty much nasty. It's very pungent. Best thing to do is add the drops in a glass filled with one or two ounces of water and take it down like a shot of tequila. And you may need the lemon wedge chaser. FYI.

Chamomile

Chamomile has been used for years as a natural sleep aide. Its calming effects not only help combat insomnia, but in even small doses it can help alleviate anxiety. What's great about this delicious, fragrant flower is that the results are quick. So if you're an immediate gratification kinda gal, this is for you! Unlike many other natural sleep aides, you do not need to ingest chamomile for weeks on end to reap the benefits. One cup of tea 45 minutes before bed should have you sleeping soundly! Chrysin, the active flavonoid component found in chamomile, is the goddess chemical that makes this baby chill you out and promotes sleepiness. Research shows that chamomile can significantly reduce the amount of time it takes to fall asleep, exhibiting almost hypnotic effects. Not only will its beauty-sleep-promoting properties make you look all fresh, rejuvenated, bright-eyed and bushy-tailed in the morning, but its antioxidant, anti-inflammatory and antiseptic properties reduce puffiness, skin inflammations, and irritations such as acne, rashes, psoriasis and eczema. Plus, it has cell-regenerating properties, which, coupled with the cell-regenerating benefits of sleep, means you'll be looking sexy hot forever.

Another reason we don't get good quality sleep at night is indigestion. As great as our intentions are to go to sleep on an empty stomach, without eating *anything* three hours before bed, don't even pretend you never hover in front of an open fridge, wearing your pjs and trying to decide what you're going to nosh on right before jumping in the sack. It happens. And you know what else happens? Indigestion and poor quality sleep. Here's where chamomile comes to the rescue. Not only will it help you sleep better, chamomile is an awesome remedy for intestinal health and indigestion. No, it won't solve the problem of eating right before bed. Your body can't easily digest food while lying horizontally, and you just won't sleep well. But if you replace that bedtime snack with a cup of chamomile tea, you'll help alleviate any discomfort, heartburn or indigestion from foods eaten earlier in the day.

HOW TO USE: Chamomile is best consumed as a tea before bed, or anytime during the day to promote relaxation. Steep two or three tablespoons in one cup of boiling water for five to ten minutes. You can also add a couple of drops of passionflower for additional anti-anxiety and sleep-promoting benefits. Other options are to add two milliliters of chamomile extract to a cup of warm water, drizzle drops of chamomile essential oil on your pillow or add a sachet of the dried flower under your pillow at night. You can also use the tea topically as skin toner and to alleviate skin irritations.

> BONUS: Researchers at the University of Southampton show that those who slept in a room infused with the scent of lavender reported a better night's sleep and woke up feeling much more energized in the morning. Sprinkle a few drops of lavender essential oil on your pillow at night, add lavender essential oil to almond oil and apply as a skin moisturizer, or soak in a warm bath infused with lavender essential oil before bed and you'll be guaranteed to have sweet dreams.

Lemon Balm

Lemon balm is a wonderfully fresh, fragrant herb that can help replace your stress-head with clear, happy thoughts. Lemon balm is a calming herb, very similar to mint and belonging to the same family. Native to the Mediterranean region of Europe and now grown in many parts of the world, lemon balm is not only a culinary ingredient but also has antibacterial, antiviral and mild sedative properties. Studies show that lemon balm's anti-anxiety properties work best as a sleep aid when combined with other sleep-inducing herbs, such as valerian, chamomile or hops. Lemon balm also contains the chemical compound eugenol, which helps calm muscle spasms and promote relaxation.

HOW TO USE: Lemon balm smells and tastes amazing, so use it whenever you can! It can be used in many dishes as a fresh or dry herb and adds a nice twist as a mint replacement in many dishes. To get the most bang out of this dainty little herb, the dried herb can be steeped into a tea, or the extract can be added to hot water or another variety of herbal tea, such as chamomile or passionflower. Soon you'll be drifting off and putting your anxiety to rest!

Oats

Yes, that's right. Your healthy breakfast staple can help put you to sleep. This complex carbohydrate is also rich in protein, in particular, tryptophan (the same amino acid found in turkey that makes us sleepy after Thanksgiving dinner!). Tryptophan is an essential (meaning you must get it from food) amino acid that, in the presence of vitamin B6 and magnesium, is responsible for the production of our feel-good transmitter, serotonin. Not only does serotonin help alleviate depression (see chapter 5), it also regulates the onset of sleep and is a precursor to melatonin production.

Oats contain the dynamic duo of tryptophan and its faithful sidekick, carbs. Here's how it works. Amino acids don't play well together — they're like a rowdy bunch of children screaming "Pick me! Pick me!" They compete for uptake into the blood stream during the digestive process, and tryptophan is just one of these amino acids trying to get your attention. So that's where carbs come in, giving tryptophan the edge. Carbs trigger the release of insulin, which pushes all the large neutral branch-chained amino acids directly into muscle cells — except for tryptophan, leaving it all by its lonesome self. But that's a good thing. Insulin pushes out all competition giving tryptophan a clear playing field to quickly cross the blood-brain barrier, get converted to serotonin, then metabolized into melatonin — which makes you feel oh-so-peaceful and relaxed, and blissfully oblivious to the amino acid bullying that just went on in your body. So, regarding your turkey dinner… it isn't just the turkey that gives you food coma, it's all the carbs you consume alongside your turkey that really knock you out!

Oats are also are a high source of vitamin B6, which is essential for the conversion of tryptophan into serotonin. B-vitamins also help reduce stress and support the adrenal glands. And, no surprise here, oats are rich in fibre, giving a feeling of fullness without all the extra calories. They're also great for digestive health, they keep you regular and also help to lower cholesterol levels.

HOW TO USE: Cook up some steel cut oats and sprinkle with cinnamon. You can have them for breakfast or have a small serving a few hours before bed as a relaxing snack. Try slicing up some apples and baking them with a little bit of water, cinnamon and oats. They also make great cookies as a healthy post-meal snack (check out my recipe on page 171). You can stir oats into yogurt instead of granola, or even use oats in soup — a different take on your traditional mushroom barley soup!

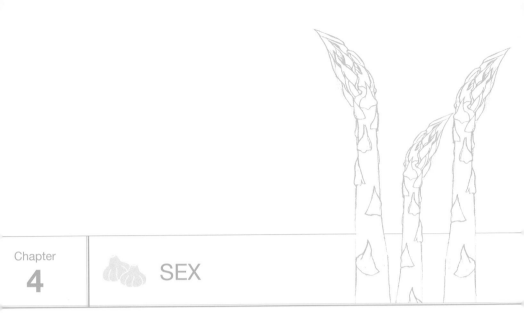

<table>
<tr><td>Chapter
4</td><td></td><td>SEX</td></tr>
</table>

Let's talk about sex. Can you believe that nearly 40 per cent of us complain of having a low sex drive? Isn't that insane? Crazy! And if you skipped straight to this chapter, then maybe you can! Low libido is the most common sexual issue among women and men. And yet healthy, regular sex is essential for optimal health and for your relationship with your partner. Fortunately, I have some secrets that can help you get in the mood!

Why sex is so important for your health
Seriously peeps. Want to achieve optimum health? Then bust out your inner sex vixen and get busy. And no, once a month — or even once a week — does not cut it. I'm talking frequent sex. The benefits reach far beyond euphoria. Not only do regular romps increase your self-confidence and emotional connection, but having sex more than once a week can also boost your immune system. Research shows that those who have frequent, safe sex have higher levels of the antibody immunoglobulin A (IgA), which helps to prevent against colds. Not only that, but sex can also boost cardiovascular health. So don't worry about giving someone a heart attack in the sack. Get wild and crazy. Having sex twice or more a week can lower blood pressure and cut the risk of heart attacks for men by HALF, versus having sex less than once a month. Also for men, having frequent ejaculations (more than 21 per month) significantly cuts the risk of prostate cancer. Got a headache? Shitty excuse. Having sex may actually help alleviate the pain — and the same goes for joint pain, muscle pain and PMS. Basically, as endorphins are increased, our levels of pain decrease. Win-win.

If all these health benefits still aren't enough motivation for you to get your sex on, you're not alone. In an iVillage survey of 2,000 women, 63 per cent of them said they would rather sleep, watch a movie or read than have sex. Seriously people, that's almost two-thirds of women! And on the flip side, a good chunk of men also suffer from sexual problems such as erectile dysfunction or premature ejaculation. What gives? Work and family demands, everyday stress, certain medications and health issues can cause sexual desire to plummet faster than a sinking ship, leaving you and your partner frustrated. But before you go running out the door to grab a prescription for Cialis, first check out these key libido-boosting nutrients to help get you and your partner in the mood.

Zinc

One of the many causes of low sex drive in both men and women is a decline in testosterone, the most important libido-boosting sex hormone. A poor diet high in saturated fats, caffeine and alcohol can result in this. On the flip side, a healthy diet and lifestyle can help balance hormones and naturally boost testosterone, whetting your appetite for sex. One of the most important testosterone-boosting nutrients is zinc. Zinc is essential for testosterone production and sperm production, and it blocks the enzyme that converts testosterone into estrogen. Low levels of zinc correlate to erectile and sexual dysfunction.

> Foods high in zinc: Oysters, lobster, Crab, Wheat germ, Sesame seeds, Roasted pumpkin seeds, Crimini mushrooms, Spinach, Summer squash, Cocoa powder, Miso , Maple syrup.

Tyrosine

Tyrosine stimulates the production of dopamine, which is our neurotransmitter responsible for pleasure and arousal. It's the core of our sexual drive and motivation. It stimulates our reward center, guilty pleasures and desires. It drives and motivates us to do things. The pleasure/reward associated with sex is typically driven by dopamine. Hence, low levels of dopamine can weaken our desire to have sex. Foods rich in the amino acid tyrosine can stimulate dopamine production, as tyrosine converts to dopamine in the brain. Tyrosine can either be obtained though food, or can be manufactured in the body as the result of the conversion of the amino acid phenylalanine.

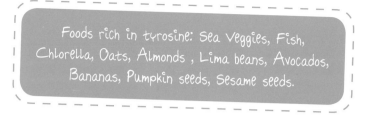

Foods rich in tyrosine: Sea Veggies, Fish, Chlorella, Oats, Almonds , Lima beans, Avocados, Bananas, Pumpkin seeds, Sesame seeds.

HEART-HEALTHY NUTRIENTS

Here's the deal. If you want to enjoy sex, you need blood flowing to your genitals, pronto. In women, an increase in genital blood flow induces vaginal swelling and spurs the lubrication process. In men, blood vessels in the penis dilate, fill with blood and cause an erection. Now, what do you think happens if there's a build-up of plaque in the arteries? Blood wouldn't flow freely, now would it? A reduction in blood flow means less blood pumping to the genitals. Therefore, high cholesterol is directly correlated to erectile dysfunction. So if all the other reasons to embrace a heart-healthy diet were not enough motivation, maybe an improved sex life will be! Omega-3s play a star role here, as they lower blood triglyceride levels by 25 to 45 per cent, and also boost dopamine levels in the pleasure centre of the brain. Here are some other nutrients that can get your blood flowing:

L-arginine is an essential amino acid that stimulates the release of nitric oxide from the walls of blood vessels, dilating the blood vessels and improving blood flow. Pretty much the same deal as Viagra.

Vitamin B3 (niacin) is essential for circulation and improved blood flow, especially to your extremities. It also increases the skin's sensitivity to touch. Fun times!

Vitamin B6 helps with the conversion of neurotransmitters and increases blood flow, meaning it can help boost dopamine levels, transitioning you from disinterested damsel to a purring sex-kitten.

Vitamin E aids in the production of sex hormones, supplies the genitals with oxygen and protects against free-radical damage.

Selenium is a mineral essential for a man's sex drive and sperm production. Half the selenium in a man's body is found in his testicles!

Health Tip for your man: Selenium is a mineral essential for a man's sex drive and sperm production. Half the selenium in a man's body is found in his testicles. Toss him a couple of Brazil nuts to keep him pumped (literally).

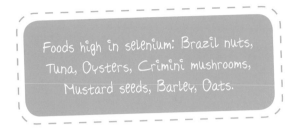

Foods high in selenium: Brazil nuts, Tuna, Oysters, Crimini mushrooms, Mustard seeds, Barley, Oats.

SEXY FOODS

Maca

Maca is known as "nature's Viagra," so if you want a natural way to increase your libido, this is the superfood for you! A little bit of maca in your system and you'll be raring to go!

While touted for its sex-enhancing properties, maca does much more than increase libido. This powerhouse Peruvian herb is packed with nutrients and has been used for centuries to increase energy, improve memory and concentration, overcome anemia and fight depression. Those ancient Peruvians knew what they were talking about! Maca is an adaptogen, meaning it helps restore balance within the entire body system. One of nature's greatest aphrodisiacs, maca is known to increase sex drive, stamina, performance and frequency! It also has claims to increase erectile function and sperm count in men, as well as the ovarian function in women, enhancing fertility. It does this by improving overall health, vitality, energy and balance, naturally increasing libido.

One of the best qualities of maca is its ability to support the body's endocrine system. Maca on its own does not contain hormones, nor does it actually change blood hormone levels when ingested. Rather, it restores the endocrine system through the hypothalamus pituitary axis by improving communication between the brain and the pituitary gland, as well as the adrenals. This ensures proper hormone balancing and secretion within the body. So basically, it helps ensure the message of whatever hormone is actually required gets across.

For example, let's say you had a craving for vanilla ice cream and you asked your man to get some it for you, but (like most men) he wasn't really listening. So one of two things happens: either he doesn't bring you ice cream at all (because he wasn't listening) or he brings you chocolate instead. The end result is that, you don't get what you want and you're not happy. Fail. But, if you both took maca, there would be great communication between the two of you, he would get your message clearly, would bring you vanilla ice cream and all would be good! Maca just improves the pituitary glands' "listening skills" to send and receive the correct info, without changing blood hormone levels. Too bad maca doesn't work on relationships! From a 'speaking and listening' perspective, that is. On the sex front, it's got your back!

The maca root is also a rich source of energy-dense complex carbohydrates and packs in more than 10 per cent protein, including 19 amino acids. It's also super-high in B-vitamins (particularly B1 and B2, which help to boost energy and manage stress, respectively), vitamins C and E, and a plethora of minerals, including significant amounts of iron (more than most red meats, beans, seeds and nuts), potassium, magnesium, zinc, iodine and calcium. Got milk? No need when maca trumps milk gram for gram in the amount of calcium. Maca is also a significant source of dietary fibre and essential fatty acids. How sexy is that?

Maca's medicinal use dates back to Incan civilization as early as 1600 B.C., and it is still commonly used by Peruvians as both a food and herbal remedy to increase fertility, mood, stamina and endurance. While the long list of benefits is impressive, here are a few really worth noting:

- Increases energy, stamina and athletic performance
- Improves memory, concentration and mental alertness
- Alleviates depression and enhances mood
- Reduces symptoms of menopause and PMS
- Balances endocrine system, hormones and thyroid function
- Natural aphrodisiac
- Enhances sexual function in both men and women
- Helps fight anemia with its concentrated source of iron (higher than most red meats!)
- Improves bone health through high levels of calcium and magnesium

HOW TO USE: Maca can be mixed into your breakfast cereals, blended into your smoothies or can be used to substitute a portion of the flour ingredient in baked goods such as cakes and cookies. If you are making a cake, replace up to a quarter to half of the flour with maca powder and you'll give a whole new meaning to devil's food cake (wink, wink).

Pumpkin seeds

These delicious seeds, sometimes called pepitas, are rich in B-vitamins, vitamin E, zinc and essential fatty acids, including oleic acids, omega-6 and the anti-inflammatory, antioxidant omega-3.

For men, these seeds help support prostate health due to their high magnesium and zinc properties. As men age, their levels of zinc tend to decline, which can lead to testosterone deficiency, erectile dysfunction and enlargement of the prostate. Zinc can help reduce prostate inflammation and is essential in building seminal fluid and increasing sperm count. These seeds are rich in phytosterols, which also contribute to prostate health. They have also been praised for their cholesterol-lowering properties. And as we know, the higher the cholesterol, the weaker the erection!

In women, these nutrient-rich seeds help build hormones, activate sexual organs and increase sexual fluid secretions. They also contain the amino acid myosin, which is essential for muscle contractions. And if you want to reap the benefits of good sex, you might want to ensure those muscles are in good working order for the big O!

HOW TO USE: Pumpkin seeds should be eaten raw (not roasted) to maintain all their health benefits. They can be eaten on their own as a crunchy snack, combined with other nuts and seeds, added to trail mix, topped on salads, cereals and oatmeal, or sprinkled on soups for added texture and crunch. You can also enjoy their health benefits by drizzling pumpkin seed oil on veggies or using raw pumpkin seed butter as a spread. Soaking the raw seeds for eight to 12 hours prior to eating makes them easier to digest. They can then be dehydrated to restore crunch, while still maintaining their nutritional benefits.

Garlic

Although garlic may seem like the antithesis of sexiness, pop back a few mints, suck on some cinnamon sticks and spice up your sex life with this potent alliaceae bad-boy. Yep, garlic will get your blood flowing in all the right places. Garlic contains allicin, which is the sulfur-based organic compound that gives garlic its funky order. Well, start to love it, because it's allicin that increases blood flow to sexual organs. It does this by increasing nitric oxide, which is a chemical gas used by blood vessel walls to trigger the arteries and surrounding muscles, causing them to relax. The more nitric oxide, the wider the blood vessels become and the greater the increase in blood flow, causing a sexual response in both males and females. Viagra knocks off this process through its chemically-created blue pill that enhances nitric oxide pathways in the penis, triggering an erection.

In addition, garlic also helps prevent blood platelets from building up and forming artery-clogging blood clots, which assists the whole blood flow process. A study published in the *Journal of Nutrition* concluded that garlic, coupled with an increase in dietary protein, increases testicular testosterone (the sex hormone). Garlic is also a great natural antibiotic and has anti-bacterial and anti-fungal properties, and can help protect against some cancers.

HOW TO USE: Minced, chopped, crushed, smashed. That's how allicin is formed and becomes effective. When alliin, which is the preceding compound in garlic, is combined with the garlic's own enzyme (alliinase) it converts to allicin. The only way the enzymes can break down alliin into allicin is through this manual chopping process, or through some serious chewing. On its own, alliin does not contain any beneficial health properties. It must be converted into allicin in order to be effective. It also takes some time for this process to occur, so after you've minced your garlic, let it sit for a few minutes to allow time for the magic to happen. It is best to eat garlic raw, as heat destroys allicin. Cooking a garlic whole can kill the enzymes before allicin is formed, making it pretty much worthless. Add some minced, raw garlic to salad dressings, mix with extra virgin olive oil and drizzle over steamed veggies… perhaps some asparagus!

Asparagus
Just look at the darn thing — it looks phallic! Now get your mind out of the gutter and get a hold of these sex-boosting facts. Asparagus is super-high in vitamin E, which is essential for a healthy sex drive. Vitamin E helps to increase vaginal lubrication and can help increase energy and stamina. Its powerful antioxidant properties help protect sex cell membranes and oxygen-rich blood flow to the genitals from free-radical damage. It also aids in the dilation of blood vessels, increasing blood and oxygen flow.

Asparagus is high in niacin (vitamin B3), which also helps enlarge blood vessels and produce sex hormones. In addition, niacin is required for histamine production, which is absolutely necessary for orgasm. It also increases the skin's sensitivity to touch and produces that "sexual flush," making the whole experience much more pleasurable. Asparagus is also a good source of vitamin B6, which ignites our feel-good transmitters; zinc to enhance libido-boosting testosterone; and selenium, which helps increase sperm count. It's also rich in antioxidant, immune-boosting and beautifying vitamin C, keeping us at the top of our game.

HOW TO USE: Asparagus is super versatile whether you're looking for a snack or an addition to a great meal. Try raw and chop into your fave salad or dip with hummus. Steam some up and toss with hemp or olive oil, sea salt and a squeeze of lemon. Or through into your next stir fry or soup.

Walnuts
Walnuts have been alive and kicking for more than 2,000 years. They were commonly used as an aphrodisiac in Roman times, and you'll be happy to hear they are still used for this same purpose today. Throughout history, these nutritious nuts have been linked to love and fertility, and for good reason.

Walnuts are very high in a wide range of nutrients that support not only sexual and reproductive health, but also the health of many other body systems. Besides being high in protein and a great source of beneficial fibre, there are several reasons walnuts are associated with sex and love. Walnuts are a good source of folic acid, an important nutrient for women who are trying to conceive. They also contain L-arginine, which, apart from being an essential amino acid in the body, helps men attain erection and maintain stamina in bed. But don't worry, L-arginine is an equal opportunity nutrient — it increases libido and intensifies sexual sensation in women too.

Walnuts and walnut oil are a great source of omega-3 fatty acids. Diets that include these healthy fats stimulate the fire necessary to sustain a healthy sex life. Healthy fats are essential for lovers because they are necessary for the production of many sex hormones. Walnuts also contain zinc. Both zinc and omega-3s are great for the sexual health of men, supporting heart and blood circulation. Research shows that walnuts are directly linked to helping some men maintain erections. Walnuts can increase sex drive so substantially that in recent years they have been used in an alternative form of Viagra. You might want to mix these into your husband's breakfast cereal in the morning!

L-tyrosine, which is the precursor to dopamine, is another amino acid found in walnuts that helps boost your sex drive. Dopamine is the neurotransmitter that will get you begging for it! It stimulates motivation, drive and the reward/pleasure center of your brain. But settle down cowgirl — that's not all — walnuts are rich in vitamin E, which not only helps balance hormones, naturally stimulating your libido, but also makes your skin super soft, begging for it to be touched!

HOW TO USE: Like all other nuts, they are best enjoyed raw. And feel free to throw them in wherever you like — enjoy them alone as a snack, ground into a pie crust, tossed into a salad, stirred into yogurt, blended into smoothies and mixed into breakfast cereals. Walnut oil not only makes a great salad dressing, but also a skin moisturizer… and edible massage oil! These nuts are calorie-dense, so consume only a small handful a couple of times a week to reap the rewards of a healthy and happy sex life.

Sacha inchi seeds

When it comes to Omega-3 and sex, O-M-G! The richest source of plant-based Omega-3 on the planet, sacha inchi seeds (aka SaviSeed) are a must in your diet if you're looking for more lovin'. The reason: Omega-3 fatty acids are vital to cardiovascular health aiding in the reduction of arterial plaque and improving the health of your heart. The healthier your heart and arteries, the greater the blood flow throughout your body – including your genitals. The greater the blood flow to the genitals, the greater… well… ya know! Even more on the other health benefits of sacha inchi on page 52.

HOW TO USE: This aphrodisiac seed is available as a bite-size snack or oil. The oil can be used in salad dressings, sauces or drizzled on your favorite dish. The seeds make a great snack or add-on for salads, cereals or yogurts. They have a nutty flavor so I've found they make a great base for sauces and dips too. You can also find SaviSeeds chocolate and caramel coated for a more indulgent, yet still healthy treat. If you really want to get your sex on, you must try my Luv Drunk Pears dessert recipe on page 183. It'll have you falling in love all over again!

DEPRESSION

It is estimated that in the next 10 years depression will be the second-most common health problem in the world, with women being affected almost twice as much as men. Most of us occasionally feel sad or down for many reasons, such as the loss of a loved one, the end of a relationship or losing a job. However, for many, this overall feeling of sadness can last beyond weeks. It can be debilitating, affecting work performance, relationships and social interactions. It can create a feeling of hopelessness, pessimism, low self-esteem and withdrawal. It can cause fatigue, exhaustion and lack of motivation to do anything. Unfortunately, many people who feel this way think it's the norm. That it's uncontrollable. That it's just "how they are." This is not the case! You don't need to feel that way. Depression is not just a "feeling" of unhappiness. It is an ailment that affects the mind, just like the flu or arthritis affects the body. And, like the flu, it can be prevented and treated. If you think you are struggling with something more serious than everyday blues, it is best to consult with your health practitioner or psychotherapist, as he or she can best help you. Depression *is* treatable. You *can* feel your absolute best every day. And what you put into your body *does* make a significant difference.

Sugar, alcohol and caffeine

Depression isn't just in the mind — it involves the whole body. There are many nutritional factors that can trigger or compound depression. Stimulants such as sugar, alcohol and caffeine can create blood sugar imbalances, which can lead to depression. Too much caffeine can deplete the body of vitamin B6, the crucial nutrient required for the production of our "happy" transmitter, serotonin. As well, blood sugar imbalance (and lactose intolerance) prevents the absorption of tryptophan in the intestine, which impedes the production of dopamine and serotonin. So, if you're the type that when life throws you lemons, you'd rather use them as a twist to accompany your big bottle of Grey Goose. Or perhaps just bury yourself in that triple layer chocolate fudge cake and grande caramel macchiato, it may not help so much. Sure, we might feel fab for a whole nanosecond (or two) while all that sugar, alcohol and caffeine shocks our system, but once we come off that high, we'll feel even more like shit.

Allergies and food sensitivities

Allergies and food sensitivities can also play a major role in depression. Food allergies promote inflammation, alter hormones and brain chemicals, and can lead to both schizophrenia and one of its main symptoms, depression. In fact, in a study conducted by allergy expert Dr. William Philpott involving 52 patients with schizophrenia, 64 per cent adversely reacted to wheat, 50 per cent to cow's milk, 75 per cent to tobacco and 30 per cent to petrochemical hydrocarbons. Many allergies and food intolerances are due to artificial food dyes and pesticides, so eating natural, organic food as much as possible is essential for your physical *and* mental health!

Nutritional deficiencies

Another factor that can lead to depression is nutritional deficiency. Diets high in refined sugar, processed foods, pesticides, preservatives and additives have all been linked to depression. But it's not just the bad stuff you're adding in that's making you depressed — it's also the good stuff you're keeping out! When we fill our stomachs with foods that are nutritionally void, there's no room left for all the health-giving foods our bodies and minds crave. And depriving your body of the essential nutrients it needs for optimal health will almost certainly have a negative impact on your mental health.

Understanding serotonin: our happy neurotransmitter

Serotonin is our feel-good neurotransmitter! Although all serotonin is produced in the brain, about 20 per cent of serotonin resides in the central nervous system, where its role is to help regulate mood, sleep and appetite. It also plays a star role in helping combat depression and stimulates a feeling of overall well being, which is why it's known as the happiness hormone. The remaining 80 per cent of serotonin is found in the gut, where it helps regulate intestinal activity, as well as in blood platelets. Depression is largely associated with a serotonin deficiency. If there aren't enough serotonin neurotransmitters being sent and received, depression can strike.

Did you know? Men synthesize 52 per cent more serotonin than women, which is one of the reasons why more women become depressed than men.

Eat your antidepressants

Tryptophan, an amino acid found in foods such as sacha inchi seeds, eggs, beans, oats, chicken and turkey, is the precursor to serotonin production. With the help of vitamin B6, vitamin C and zinc, tryptophan is converted to a chemical called 5-HTP, which crosses the blood-brain barrier and converts to serotonin. Tryptophan and 5-HTP are the *only* precursors to serotonin production. Antidepressants *do not* manufacture serotonin.

With respect to serotonin, the only thing anti-depressants do is block the re-uptake of serotonin from the "sending" neuron so it's not reabsorbed. This increases circulation of serotonin in the synapse (the space between neurons) so that it can be more readily available to be picked up by a receptor site. These are called selective serotonin reuptake inhibitors (SSRIs) and include medications such as Prozac, Zoloft, Paxil, Celexa, Lexapro and Luvox.

Other anti-depressants focus on the neurotransmitters dopamine and epinephrine, which, although also linked with depression, are mainly associated with lack of motivation and energy, as opposed to serotonin, which is associated with mood.

However, none of these meds actually *manufacture* serotonin, but only rather maintain what is already existent through the foods you eat. Only changing your diet or supplementing with 5-HTP can actually increase the production of serotonin. Plus, many people can't tolerate anti-depressants due to their laundry list of side effects, such as anxiety, sexual dysfunction, weight loss or weight gain, just to name a few.

KEY NUTRIENTS THAT ALLEVIATE AND PREVENT DEPRESSION

Omega-3 fatty acids

Sixty per cent of the brain is made up of fat. We need fat for our brains to function optimally. But it's the *type* of fat that is critical. Just like trans fats are bad for your heart, the same holds true for your mind. Unhealthy fats, such as saturated and trans fats, will not only cause a plaque build-up in your arteries, but will also congest the brain. A third of brain fat is made up of polyunsaturated fatty acids (PUFAs). In turn, PUFAs are made up of omega-3 fatty acids and omega-6 fatty acids. Good sources of omega-3s include cold-water oily fish, algae, nuts and seeds such as flax, sacha inchi and chia. The optimal ratio in our diet is two parts omega-6s to one part omega-3s. However, today's North American diet has shifted the ratio to more like 20:1. This significantly skewed ratio causes inflammation, allergies, cognitive issues and a whole host of other problems. Omega-6 fatty acids promote inflammation, whereas omega-3 fatty-acids reduce inflammation. This is why we need to add more omega-3s to our diet and make a conscious effort to reduce the amount of omega-6s consumed.

Foods rich in omega-3:
Wild salmon, Mackerel,
Herring, Anchovies, Algae,
Sacha inchi seeds,
Chia seeds, Flax,
Walnuts, Hemp.

Foods rich in omega-6:
Vegetable oil, Palm oil,
Sunflower oil,
Safflower oil, Canola oil,
Soybean oil, Corn oil.

Omega-3 fatty acids are *the* most important fat for your brain and for alleviating depression. A Harvard study indicated that use of omega-3 fatty acids is an effective alternative to drug therapies in treating depression and when complemented with traditional drug therapies can increase their efficacy. A meta-analysis of 10 studies found that omega-3s had significant effects in treating depression, bipolar depression and ADHD.

Omega-3 fatty acids (especially DHA) stabilize the brain's cell membranes, making them more fluid and making communication across the synapses more effective. For example, imagine you are a messenger (neurotransmitter) that is trying to send a gift of happiness to your neighbour. However, there is a river separating your house from your neighbour's. Now, if this river is crystal clear and free flowing, you can get across it no problem. But if it's all swamp-like, thick and nasty, it might take you a bit longer to cross. Omega-3 fatty acids are fluid-like fats that assist in the transduction of neurotransmitters from one neuron to another. The lack of omega-3s can cause communication breakdown to occur — the message gets stuck in the swamp, so to speak. Omega-3s also help increase your brain's neuronal connections and the number of feel-good serotonin receptor sites.

B-vitamins
B-vitamins are like a whole family of superstars, just waiting to kick into action and boot your depression to the curb. B1 (thiamine) fuels the brain with glucose for energy and is required for nerve stimulation. A deficiency in B3 (niacin) is liked to both depression and anxiety. B3 is used by health professionals in the treatment of schizophrenia. Vitamin B6 is required for the production of serotonin and other neurotransmitters and essential in regulating mood. B12 is required for the production of serotonin and other neurotransmitters, and essential for the nervous system to function properly. There is a strong link between depression and a deficiency in vitamin B12.

Folate
Folic acid isn't just for women who are preggers! Folate deficiency is common in

those with depression. Folate is another nutrient required for the production of serotonin. So if you're lacking in folate, you're probably lacking in serotonin, which we know can lead to depression. Good sources of folate (other than prenatal vitamins!) include spinach, broccoli, lentils, asparagus and bananas.

Do you know the difference between folate and folic acid? Folate is naturally produced within your body, folic acid is a dietary/supplemental form of folate.

FOODS THAT FIGHT DEPRESSION

Fish oil and/or cold-water oily fish (wild salmon)

EPA and DHA are derivatives of omega-3 fatty acids. They can be found naturally in oily fish such as salmon, tuna, halibut, herring and cod. When choosing a fish oil, keep in mind that it should contain significantly more EPA than DHA, and deliver no less than 1,000 milligrams of EPA per day for adults and 500 to 600 milligrams of EPA per day for children. EPA and DHA can also be converted in the body from ALA (alpha linolenic acids), which are found in plant-based sources such as nuts and seeds. However, the conversion rate from ALA to EPA and DHA in humans is fairly low, which is why direct, fish-based sources of EPA and DHA are most effective for the treatment of depression. For example, someone who eats fish once every two weeks would get the same amount of EPA as someone who consumes over three tablespoons of flax seed oil (source of ALA) every day.

TIP: Fish oil is also phenomenal for cardiovascular heath. Fish oil lowers triglycerides by 25 to 45 per cent and also raises HDL, a good cholesterol, by five to 15 per cent.

HOW TO USE: Look for a fish oil with at least 1,000 milligrams of EPA per daily dosage. Be sure to purchase oil in capsule form instead of liquid. Liquid fish oils become rancid very quickly. They are fine until they are opened, but once they are opened they oxidize rapidly, even if kept in the fridge. They are extremely sensitive to light, heat and oxygen, so every time you open and close the bottle, it will be exposed to oxygen and the oil will be damaged. Also ensure you are using pharmaceutical grade oil — if not, you may be ingesting more than you bargained for, including contaminants such as heavy metals! Not so good for the brain.

Sacha inchi

Although sometimes coined as an Inca peanut, there's nuttin' nutty about this seed. Yep, that's right, sacha inchi is a seed, not a nut, and can also go by the names SaviSeed, sacha peanut, mountain peanut, and, plukenetia volubilis (for the grown-up, scientific types). The seeds are found in the plush, star-shaped green fruit of the semi-perennial, shrub-like, viney sacha inchi plant that grows deep within the Peruvian Amazon rainforest. The incubation combination of intense sunlight and mineral-rich soil contributes to its kick-ass nutritional density.

Sacha inchi seeds are one of the most nutrient-dense seeds around, especially when it comes to brain health. At approximately 48 per cent, these seeds contain the highest plant-based source of omega-3 fatty acids in the world! Even those these seeds are a plant-based source of omega-3s, because they contain such a concentrated amount, even with a low conversion to DHA, they still come out on top. This helps improve cognitive functioning and fight depression by improving the reception of our lovely mood-lifting neurotransmitter serotonin. In addition, these omega-3 fatty acids are significant in helping lower bad cholesterol, improving overall heart heath. Sacha inchi seeds have strong anti-inflammatory properties, which ward off pain and disease. The seeds are also high in fibre, which binds onto cholesterol (helping your body to eliminate it), helps to improve digestive health, increases satiety, and helps to balance blood sugar levels, which is paramount in combating depression.

And, at almost 28 per cent, these seeds are also extremely high in digestible protein. Ounce for ounce, they trump any meat source of protein — and most other seeds! And why should this make you happy (literally)? For every gram of protein, sacha inchi seeds have 29 milligrams of serotonin-making tryptophan. What's important here is the ratio of tryptophan to total protein. Remember, amino acids compete, so the greater the ratio of tryptophan as a percentage of protein, the more clout it has relative to the other amino acids, increasing its odds of being able to work its magic. To put things into perspective, check out the chart below:

	Total Protein /100G	Total Tryptophan /100G	% Tryptophan /100G
Sacha Inchi	28	0.812	2.90%
Egg Whites	10.9	0.125	1.15%
Turkey	21.89	0.243	1.11%
Sesame Seeds	17	0.370	2.17%
Milk	3.22	0.080	2.34%
Spirulina	57.47	0.930	1.62%

We usually associate tryptophan with turkey, right? Well, not so much. Not only do sacha inchi seeds have more total protein than turkey, ounce for ounce, they have over three times the amount of tryptophan. Plus, the ratio of tryptophan as a percentage of total protein significantly trumps the big bird.

In addition to its happiness-boosting properties, the seed's rich protein content combined with the anti-inflammatory omega-3 make it ideal for a great snack to aid in quick muscle recovery and growth. It's also high in iodine, which is good for thyroid function and metabolism, and a great source of the antioxidant vitamins A and E, which are great for improving skin and hair!

HOW TO USE: Sacha inchi oil can be used cold, drizzled on veggies, mixed into salad dressings or stirred into blended smoothies. The seeds can be added to a trail mix combined with other nuts, seeds and dried fruit, can be used as a topper for salads, cereals, yogurts and other prepared dishes, or enjoyed on their own as a delicious snack! What if you want to indulge without the bulge? You're in for a treat! Sacha inchi seeds come "karma"lized and cocoa-kissed, which is the hip and "savi" new take on the old faves of beer nuts and chocolate covered almonds, which are now SO 2000-and-late. BONUS: the tiny amount of sweetness that hugs these scrumptious seeds helps increase the rate at which tryptophan enters the blood-brain barrier, speeding up the rate of serotonin production and ultimate happiness. That's right, jump for joy… it has that effect!

Saffron

Saffron is an aromatic spice native to Southwestern Asia and a culinary staple in many Middle Eastern and Indian delish dishes. Saffron comes from the dried stigma of the *crocus sativus* (saffron crocus) flower, which is a lily-like perennial. While we may tend to savour the spice in small quantities due to its high price tag, we may actually be getting more bang for our buck than we could have imagined!

Studies show that saffron works just as effectively as Prozac (an SSRI) in treating mild to moderate depression — without the side effects! Researchers at the Tehran University of Medical Sciences found that during an eight-week trial involving 40 depressed patients, 30 milligrams of saffron extract per day worked as well as 20 milligrams of Prozac per day. In another six-week study, 30 milligrams of saffron per day was compared to 100 milligrams of imipramine, a tricyclic anti-depressant. Out of 30 depressed patients, both treatments provided similar relief; however, those who took saffron didn't have the associated side effects such as dry mouth and sedation.

Crocin and safranal are two chemical compounds found in saffron that are reported to relieve depression by raising serotonin and other mood-enhancing chemicals in the brain. Crocin is a carotenoid antioxidant that gives saffron its orange colour, while safranal gives the spice its distinctive aroma. Soaking saffron before use helps to activate its mood-boosting properties. In addition to saffron's ability to bust you out of a rut, it also has anti-cancer, anti-mutagenic and antioxidant properties, helping to prevent disease. Persians have used it for years to help alleviate stomachaches, vomiting, inflammation and symptoms of PMS — which can benefit everyone! Recent research also suggests it can help boost memory. It might be worth it to break the bank and invest in some saffron — who says money can't buy happiness?

HOW TO USE: Saffron can be added to flavour rice dishes and is commonly used in Middle Eastern dishes. It can also be taken as an extract for greater therapeutic benefits. Saffron can begin to oxidize in the presence of light and oxygen, so it's best to store it in a dark container.

Brazil nuts

As the name might imply, these rich and creamy nuts are native to Brazil, as well as other South American countries such as Bolivia, Venezuela, Colombia and Peru. The trees are large and can grow to 200 feet tall, and it isn't until they're about 12 years old that they start to produce fruit. And since these fruits are more high-maintenance than a Hollywood starlet, they'll only bloom in the most pristine growing conditions. Trees that grow in the ghetto part of the rainforest get no love — the pollinating bees just don't fly there! The Brazil nut fruit resembles the fuzzy brown coconut in shape and size and houses anywhere between eight to 24 Brazil nuts.

Brazil nuts' mood-boosting properties are highly attributable to their rich selenium content. Selenium is a trace mineral and antioxidant essential to combating depression, and at roughly 100 micrograms per nut, these nuts contain the richest known source. Low selenium levels in the diet can lead to irritability, depression and fatigue. In a study conducted by Brenton and Cook in the UK, 50 subjects received 100 micrograms of selenium or a placebo every day over a five week period. The selenium intake was associated with increased mood and lower feelings of depression, anxiety and fatigue.

In addition, selenium is required for the synthesis and metabolism of thyroid hormones, which can also tamper with your mood. Those suffering from a sluggish thyroid (see chapter 8) tend to also suffer from feelings of depression and fatigue. Thyroid disease can also interrupt neurotransmitter receptor cells in the brain, preventing the feel-good chemicals from latching on. Selenium actively increases thyroid hormone T3 (triiodothyronine) by kick-starting the conversion of T4 (thyroxine), boosting metabolism and mood and helping to alleviate symptoms of thyroid disease. Selenium will make you feel good in other ways, too! It's known to boost libido, which can get you out of the dumps and into the sack! It also can help prevent cancer, especially breast and prostate cancers.

Brazil nuts house the perfect dosage of selenium. All you need is to pop one or two nuts a day to get just the right the amount of selenium (100 to 200 micrograms) to give your thyroid a boost and your brain a pick-me-up. But remember to stop there. Anymore and not only will the excess calories tip the scale, but too much selenium can become toxic, especially when pushing the threshold of 3,200 micrograms.

Brazil nuts are rich in vitamin B1 (thiamin), which helps stabilize blood sugar levels by converting blood sugar to energy. You know how cranky and tired you get when your blood sugar plummets? The B1 in Brazil nuts prevent helps prevent these feelings of depression and fatigue. It's also essential in the production of the neurotransmitter acetylcholine, which boosts mood and improves memory. Brazil nuts are also a rich source of the antioxidant vitamin E and contribute to heart heath with their monounsaturated fats. Their higher, healthy fat content also increases satiety, keeping you fuller longer. And if you're feeling full, you're less likely to reach for those double-chocolate-chip cookies as a pick-me-up!

HOW TO USE: Enjoy one or two Brazil nuts on their own as a delicious, mood-boosting snack. Grind some up and sprinkle on oatmeal, salads, veggies or cauliflower mash, or use the ground nuts as a crust for your fish. Soak Brazil nuts overnight in water, rinse the next day and add to a blender with fresh water, then squeeze through a mesh cloth to make rich and delish Brazil nut milk. Add a thin layer of Brazil nut butter to toast or blend it into your favourite smoothie. Happiness to follow.

Spinach

Everybody knows that eating your vegetables is an important part of any healthy diet, but greens of the dark leafy variety have really upped the ante in terms of their benefits to health and the nervous system in particular. For the purposes of balancing mood, it is especially important to increase consumption of dark leafy greens like spinach.

Spinach is packed with B-vitamins, which are essential for balancing mood and keeping the nervous system in check. Low levels of folate (or B9) are directly linked to depression. In fact, folate is critical for stable moods and maintaining proper nervous system function — making it a great remedy for wild mood swings associated with PMS or other times when we feel like we're goin' a little crazy.

Dark leafy greens such as spinach, kale, collard greens and broccoli are also high in magnesium, calcium, potassium and vitamin C. These nutrients are all essential for proper nervous function and are depleted when stress is high — which is just when you need them the most! Magnesium is crucial for a healthy nervous system, and spinach provides lots of it, with just one cup containing about half of the recommended daily intake. Magnesium relaxes the body and the muscles, and a deficiency of this chillax'n nutrient is believed to be one of the causes of depression. Magnesium is involved in hundreds of important metabolic functions, and a large portion of current Western society is believed to be deficient. So get munching on those leafy greens, people!

Spinach and other leafy greens also contain tryptophan, which converts to serotonin in the body, enabling us to feel happy. Tryptophan can only be obtained through diet, and leafy greens like spinach are some of the best whole food sources.

HOW TO USE: Spinach is best consumed either raw or lightly steamed, as other methods of cooking can drain key nutrients, including all those mentioned that are essential for mood support. Have a crisp spinach salad for lunch or even blend some leaves into your smoothie — you won't taste the greens, but your body will feel them!

FOOD-WEIGHT CONNECTION

Discover the top nutrients and foods to help keep muffin tops and man boobs at bay!

FOOD—WEIGHT CONNECTION

You get up early for a run, watch Oprah on the elliptical, take the stairs instead of the elevator, eat clean, avoid sugars and nix extra calories, but you still aren't dropping the pounds. Frustrated, yet unwilling to give up on those barely-worn skinny jeans you've had in your closet for years now, you decide to pull yourself together and opt for a plain ol' salad with dressing on the side at your next meal. As you sit there gnawing on your lettuce, out comes this perky, skinny little thing behind you and orders a burger without a flinch of guilt. What's up with that?

Before you decide to take her out and whip your untouched vinaigrette at her scrawny ass (read Section 1 on how food affects your mood), know this: The difference between the two of you is not necessarily the calories you consume, but *how your body responds to the calories you consume*.

Before we dive further into how the food you eat can affect your metabolism, I want to shed some light on some sneaky things that could be sabotaging your weight-loss efforts.

SNEAKY SEDUCTIONS

Fat-free foods
Ever notice how many fat-free foods have been creeping up on our grocery shelves over the past several years, and yet more and more people are becoming overweight or obese? There is a direct correlation between the increase in fat-free foods and the increase in societal weight gain. North Americans are the highest consumers of fat-free foods but also have the highest rate of obesity in the world!

How fat-free foods promote fat storage

When fats are removed from foods, they are typically replaced with excess sodium, refined sugars, artificial sweeteners and chemical fillers to make the food taste good; all of which contribute to weight *gain*. These foods also tend to have the same number of calories as the fat-free versions, so your body will store any excess calories as fat anyway. And the thing is, our bodies actually need fat. Fat triggers our satiation levels and will keep us fuller longer with smaller amounts of food. Fat-free varieties don't provide the same level of satiation, causing us to eat approximately 28 per cent more calories per day. The fat isn't the problem — it's all the excess sugar that's making you fat!

Sugar

Sugars are stored in your body as stubborn *fat*! No more than 10 per cent of your daily caloric intake should come from sugars. For the average person, this can translate to around 40 to 50 grams. To put things into context, some fat-free, fruit-flavored yogurts can have up to 21 grams of sugar. One cup of 100 per cent fruit juice has 25 grams of sugar — half of our recommended daily intake!

As sugars are absorbed into your bloodstream, your blood sugar level rises. In order to lower blood sugar levels, the pancreas releases a hormone called insulin, which moves sugar from the blood into your cells, where the sugar can be used as a source of energy. The more refined the sugar, the greater stress on your pancreas, which can eventually lead to weight gain and illnesses such as diabetes.

Your body needs sugar for brain function, muscle and liver glycogen. However, excess sugar is stored in your cells as fat. Glucagon is a hormone that takes the fat out of storage and releases it so your body can burn it off. When your body is producing insulin to bring your sugar high down, it cannot produce glucagon. The result: not only are you storing extra fat, but your body has the inability to burn fat that is already stored — double fat whammy!

What's worse is that most fat-free foods contain poor-quality, highly-refined sugars such as high-fructose corn syrup. Even extremely small dosages cause tremendous negative impact to blood sugar levels — causing you to crave even *more* sugar.

Many high-sugar, fat-storing foods masquerade as "health foods" and should be avoided, including fruit juice, non-fat fruit-flavoured yogurts, breakfast cereals, high/refined-sugar granolas and sauces such as BBQ sauce, ketchup and teriyaki sauce. Here's a look at the amount of sugar in some everyday foods. I bet some will surprise you!

Food Item	Grams Sugar
Ben & Jerry's vanilla ice cream	16g
Starbucks grande latte	17g
Subway 6-inch sweet onion teriyaki chicken sandwich	17g
Pizza Hut meatball sandwich	20g
Tropicana 100% orange juice (8 oz.)	25g
Vitamin water (20 oz. bottle)	33g
Oscar Mayer Lunchables (crackers, turkey, cheese)	36g
Pizza Hut crispy chicken salad (without dressing!)	37g
Coke (1 can)	39g
Apple crisp	84g

What to do
Choose naturally fat-free foods, such as fruits and veggies, that aren't laced with chemical fillers, refined sugars and artificial sweeteners. Opt for small amounts of healthy fats, such as nuts, seeds, extra virgin olive oil and avocado. These will keep you fuller longer, causing you to eat less and delivering a much higher nutritional punch than artificially-created, fat-free foods.

Zero-calorie sweeteners
In our effort avoid sugar, we may reach for "diet" foods and drinks, thinking it will help shrink our waistline. Not so much. In fact, studies show it can actually *expand* your waistline.

How zero-calorie sweeteners promote fat storage
Studies have shown that those who drink one can of diet soda a day have a 34 per cent increase in their risk of developing metabolic syndrome and a 41 per cent increase in risk of becoming overweight and/or obese. In fact, those who drink diet soda have an even greater risk of becoming overweight or obese than the full-sugar, regular soda drinkers! How is this so? The theory is that artificial sweeteners interfere with the body's hormonal response to foods. The sweet taste tricks our body into thinking we ate something sweet, but when the calories aren't there to match up it starts to crave them — causing us to eat more sweet foods and calories to satisfy the deficit. In another study conducted by Purdue University, rats that ate yogurt sweetened with zero calorie sweeteners gained more weight and body fat. Artificial sweeteners confuse our hypothalamus. Our innate ability to detect that we've eaten enough becomes inefficient and, instead stopping when we are satiated, we just keep eating and eating and eating.

In addition, artificial sweeteners such as aspartame block the brain's production of serotonin, our feel-good neurotransmitter that also controls appetite. Low serotonin levels trigger the craving for sugar and carbs, foods that increase serotonin levels. Therefore, eating artificial sweeteners will cause us to keep craving — and eating — more sugar and carbs.

What to do

Now that you're ditching artificial sweeteners, you may still want a little sweetness from time-to-time. White or brown sugar may seem like the only options left but don't be fooled, just because they're not synthetically-produced, it doesn't mean they're good for you. Although white sugar is derived from the cane or beet plant, all the nutrients and minerals have been stripped away with nothing left but a sweet, nutritionally-void substance that is extremely high-glycemic, causing blood sugar imbalances and is a leading cause of weight gain, obesity and diabetes. Not only that, but sugar also suppresses the immune system and feeds diseases, viruses, bacteria and yeasts including candida. And brown sugar's no better; it's just white sugar with added molasses! Although it can be hard to cut out sugar completely, here are some 'better-than' alternatives to the highly-refined white stuff.

Stevia

Stevia is a natural sweetener derived from stevia leaf, an herb native to South America. It is virtually calorie-free and has no impact on blood sugar levels making it a great alternative for diabetics, those on sugar-reduced diets or those watching their weight. It is much sweeter than sugar – about 100-400 times – and can have a bitter or pungent aftertaste so a little goes a long way.

Coconut palm sugar (coconut palm nectar)

Coconut sugar is a natural sugar derived directly from the sap of the coconut tree's flower blossoms. The sap is collected, boiled and crystallized into sugar crystals. It's low on the glycemic index and puts less stress on the liver than agave nectar. It's rich in minerals – magnesium, potassium and zinc – and vitamins B and C. And it tastes DELICIOUS! Kind of like caramel or the top of creme brule!

Raw honey

Although honey is higher on the glycemic index, RAW honey (not to be confused with the processed honey found in most cupboards) is loaded nutrients. Raw honey is a thick, cloudy colour with a wax-like consistency. Raw honey has anti-microbrial properties and is rich in antioxidants, phytonutrients and enzymes.

Yacon syrup

Yacon syrup is a natural, low-calorie sweetener that actually helps to balance blood-sugar. It's made primarily of fructooligosaccharide (FOS) which acts as a prebiotic that stimulates colon health, helps increase the absorption of vitamins and improves healthy intestinal flora. FOS also helps with the absorption of calcium. It can be used as sugar or molasses substitute in recipes however you want to use less than half the amount of yacon, as it has a stronger taste.

THUTTOCKS & MAN BOOBS

That big zit you discover before a hot date. The muffin top that even your magic yoga pants can't contain. The mood swing that just sent your assistant running. All these things represent your endocrine system in action. Your endocrine system is made up of your adrenal, thyroid and pituitary glands, and is responsible for the manufacturing and distribution of hormones throughout your body. They are largely responsible for your mood, stress response, growth and development, sexual function, tissue function, hunger, fat burning, fat storage and metabolism. Even the smallest imbalance in your endocrine system can throw your body, energy, emotions and thoughts into a wicked frenzy.

WHAT IS ESTROGEN DOMINANCE?

For many, too much estrogen is a surprising cause of weight gain. Estrogens are a group of steroids acting primarily as the female sex hormone. While estrogen is an important hormone that supports reproduction and menstruation, as well as bone, cardiovascular and cognitive health, not all estrogens are created equal. There's the stronger (bad) estrogen and the weaker (good) estrogen. Our bodies make three kinds of estrogen:

- Estradiol (E2) — the strongest and most prominent estrogen. It's produced in the ovaries and plays a key role in our menstrual cycle. It also stimulates sexual desire and vaginal lubrication, increases bone health, regulates blood sugar, and supports heart health, including healthy cholesterol levels, as well as mental health. Although essential and required, too much estradiol leads to bad PMS, bloating, water retention, mood swings and weight gain (so, pretty much hell). Excess of this hormone is also linked to an increased risk of breast cancer.

- Estrone (E1) — a weaker estrogen, yet the least fave. Estrone is produced by the ovaries and adrenal glands, as well as being produced and stored in our fat cells, especially during menopause. Estrone is most prevalent in post-menopausal women. The more fat cells we have, the more estrone is produced. It can also increase the risk of breast cancer.
- Estriol (E3) — the weakest and the most fave estrogen. Estriol can block breast and uterine cells from the harmful effects of the "bad" estrogens. Estriol is dominant during pregnancy and is produced in the ovaries, in the placenta during pregnancy, as well as through the conversion of estrone and estradiol in the liver.

Estrogen isn't just a problem for the ladies in the crowd! Our bodies, both male and female, are portals of estrogen receptors, into which any type of estrogen can plug itself. The stronger the estrogen that plugs into the receptor site, the more "estrogenic" or estrogen dominant we become. This isn't a good thing. Estrogen dominance not only contributes to weight gain, but also significantly increases the incidence of uterine, endometrial and breast cancer. In fact, the National Institute of Environmental Health Sciences has listed estrogen as a known cancer-causing agent.

Thuttocks and man boobs
Excess estrogen can promote increased fat tissue in the waist, belly and other estrogen-sensitive fat tissues. For men, this is typically in the belly and chest (man boobs); for women, in the belly, lower butt and upper thighs (thuttocks), and sometimes in the back of the arms. These fats tend to be called "stubborn fat" due to their high resistance to fat burning.

The birth control pill, aging, hormone replacement therapy, steroids and excess body weight all contribute to excess estrogen. The more fat tissue a person has, the more estrogen is produced within his or her cells, which promotes more fat gain, which produces more estrogen, which promotes even more fat gain. Dang! It's no wonder we have a hard time losing weight!

In addition, certain foods and environmental factors known as endocrine-disrupting chemicals (EDCs) can actually disrupt the function of your endocrine system and the way your body uses and stores fat. All of us are exposed to estrogenic chemicals on a daily basis, many of which are capable of mimicking estrogen activity in the body.

Outside our bodies lie estrogen-mimicking chemicals. Phytoestrogens are found in some plant-based foods. Xenoestrogens are found in our environment.

Estrogen in food (phytoestrogens)

SOY, what's the deal yo?
The controversy surrounding soy can stir up more drama than an episode of Jersey Shore. While soy does have acclaimed healthy benefits, excessive amounts of highly-processed soy may have the reverse effect. Here are the deets:

Soy contains estrogen-like substances called isoflavones that mimic estrogen in the body. These isoflavones can increase the amount of estrogen that can bind onto estrogen receptors. How is this a good thing? Research suggests that since soy isoflavones are a "weaker" version of the body's regular estrogen (kind of like a cheap knock-off), they may cause less harm binding onto estrogen receptors than the stronger "bad" estrogens kicking around in your body. So some phytoestrogens like pomegranates and flax, can actually be highly beneficial in moderate quantities. But excess quantities and concentrations can lead to issues. And why settle for "not as bad" when you can kick that baby to the curb all together (see below on how).

Here's where it gets dirty. Highly-processed soy products, such as soy milk or soy cheese, have ridiculously concentrated amounts of soy isoflavones, significantly increasing the concentration of the foods' estrogenic compounds. For example, a study conducted by a New Zealand toxicologist reported that the amount of phytoestrogens in a day's worth of soy infant formula is equivalent to five birth control pills. Due to infants' tiny body weight, the impact is multiplied ten-fold. For an adult woman, two glasses of soy milk per day is enough to throw off her menstrual patterns. And really, who needs that? In addition, soy contains a compound called goitrogen, which is a thyroid-disrupting chemical. Basically, it inhibits your thyroid from absorbing iodine from the blood to manufacture and distribute hormones throughout your body, causing your metabolism to slow down. And this, as we know, puts the brakes on fat loss.

SOY, what to do? Since soy is found in over 60 per cent of packaged foods, try to limit your consumption of highly-processed soy products, such as soy milk or soy cheese, that have concentrated amounts of soy isoflavones. Instead, try to choose fermented soy products, such as miso, tempeh and soy sauce, which are healthier and easier to digest and assimilate. Also, try to increase your iodine levels when eating soy or other foods that contain goitrogens. Iodine is found in sea veggies (kelp), sea algae (chlorella), shellfish and sea salt.

Pesticides
About 90 per cent of commonly-used pesticides found in food and beverages are harmful endocrine-disrupting chemicals (EDCs). Pesticides can alter your metabolic patterns and promote fat storage, wreaking havoc on your weight loss goals. Studies show that eating an organic diet for just five days can reduce circulating pesticide EDCs to non-detectable levels.

Here are some of the worst pesticide-laden foods, which means you should choose the organic versions of these foods whenever possible: celery, peaches, strawberries, apples, blueberries, nectarines, sweet bell peppers, spinach, kale/collard greens, cherries, potatoes and imported grapes.

These foods aren't highly contaminated with pesticides, so you don't need to buy organic: onions, avocado, sweet corn, pineapples, mango, sweet peas, asparagus, kiwi fruit, cabbage, eggplant, cantaloupe, watermelon, grapefruit, sweet potatoes and honeydew melon.

Estrogen in your environment: BPAs and PVCs

All over the news, we hear about the dangers of plastics. Here's why: Bisphenol-A (BPA) and phthalates (used in making PVC), both commonly found in plastics, are compounds that mimic estrogen. Although we don't eat plastic, plastic is a common container for many of our foods and beverages, and 93 per cent of North Americans have detectable levels of BPA in our bodies!

Tips on how to avoid ingesting harmful BPAs:
1. Never heat food in plastic containers or put plastic items in the dishwasher, which can damage them and increase leaching. BPA leaches from polycarbonate sports bottles 55 times faster when exposed to boiling liquids as opposed to cold ones.
2. Never reuse a plastic container.
3. Store food in glass containers and be mindful of the lid! Some lids of glass jars are also lined with BPA-leaching plastic.
4. Cut down on canned goods, as the insides of many cans are lined with BPA plastics.

How to kick the estrogen habit

So you've been indulging in too many soy lattes and heating your lunch in the same BPA-rich plastic container for the past month but hey, now you know! What's a guy or gal to do? Here are some things you can do to remove excess estrogen from your body:

Indole-3-Carbinol/Diindolylmethane
Indole-3-Carbinol (I-3-C for non-nerds) is a chemical compound created through

the cooking and chewing of cruciferous vegetables. These include broccoli, cauliflower, Brussels sprouts, cabbage, turnips, mustard greens and kale. This compound is then broken down into diindolylmethane (DIM) in the intestinal tract and alters the metabolism of estrogen into a weaker, more beneficial version, making us less psychotic (oops — I mean estrogenic).

Calcium D-glucarate
Calcium D-glucarate is a nutrient found in fruits and vegetables, especially apples, oranges, grapefruit, broccoli, cabbage, Brussels sprouts and alfalfa. It helps to eliminate excess toxins and hormones from your body, rather than having them re-circulate back into the blood stream.

Love your liver: milk thistle and lemon water
It's important that estrogen is broken down and excreted or otherwise detoxed from the body to prevent re-absorption. The breakdown of estrogen is metabolized in the liver and passed on to bile or urine. A backed-up liver due to toxins, crap food, or partying like a rock star can put a damper on this process. Simple things like adding a few drops of milk thistle extract to your water once a day can improve its function and help eliminate toxins. Or even something as simple as starting your day with a glass of water with half a squeezed lemon can make a big difference. Take time daily to love your liver, so it can love you back!

Fibre
Fibre not only helps you feel fuller longer, it also helps to absorb and bind onto excess toxins and hormones and eliminate them from your body. Fibre is only found in plant-based foods so start noshing on whole grains, veggies and fruits.

Exercise
Since you've got that bootie, you might as well shake it! Not only is exercise sure to burn extra calories and knock off a few pounds, exercise also decreases blood estrogen levels and reduces the risk of breast cancer. One study from the US National Cancer Institute showed that exercisers who lost more than two per cent body fat had a 14 per cent reduction in estradiol levels, whereas those who lost two per cent body fat *without* exercise had no reduction in estradiol levels.

FOODS THAT COUNTERACT ESTROGEN DOMINANCE

Broccoli
Broccoli is one of those amazing superfoods that are good for just about everything. It has tremendous anti-aging benefits and is rich in antioxidants such as vitamin C, carotenoids and lutein, which protects your eyes. It's high in B-vitamins, helping to boost mood and lift depression. It's also jacked in fibre, helps protect against cardiovascular disease and has powerful antiviral,

antibacterial and anti-cancer properties. Numerous studies indicate that it protects against breast cancer and prostate cancer in particular.

Broccoli's power is drawn from dinndolylmethane (DIM). DIM is what gives the cruciferous veg its killer anti-cancer and immune-boosting properties. DIM is also what alters the metabolism of estrogen into a weaker, more beneficial form, helping reduce the severity of the bad estrogens kicking around in our body. Be sure to chew your broccoli well, as it's through mastication that DIM becomes active.

In addition, this low-cal, high-fibre rock star should be your weight loss BFF. The fibre will keep you full, without adding any extra calories. It's also rich in calcium (more absorbable calcium than milk!), which is an essential mineral for weight loss. The high fibre content coupled with the powerful detoxification properties of broccoli ensures that the bad, excess estrogen is broken down and eliminated from your body.

HOW TO USE: Bust out your steamer! You get the biggest nutritional punch from broccoli when it's steamed. Steaming broccoli breaks down the thick sulfur wall that locks in nutrients. So cooking makes it way easier for your body to absorb all the goodness this cruciferous queen has to offer. You'll need to steam broccoli until bright green and still has its crunch. If you leave it until it becomes mush, most of the nutrition will be lost. For those with thyroid imbalances, steaming broccoli also helps to break down the goitrogens which inhibit thyroid function. More on this in the next chapter... And don't forget the fat: drizzling with extra virgin olive oil or hemp seed oil increases nutrient absorption of the fat-soluble vitamins and calcium.

Green tea

Green tea is much more than just a great sushi companion. Its health benefits stem from its high levels of epigallocatechin gallate (EGCG). EGCG is a polyphenol, which is a class of phytochemicals found in high concentrations in green tea. These polyphenols are called catechins, and they give green tea its slightly bitter taste. EGCG is the dominant and most important catechin in green tea and is an extremely potent antioxidant. In fact, EGCG appears to be the most powerful of all catechins, with an antioxidant strength estimated to be from 25 to 100 times more potent than both vitamins C and E — which also contributes to its powerful anti-aging and skin-glowing benefits!

EGCG has a long list of kickass health benefits. It can help lower cholesterol levels and increase antioxidants in the blood. Studies have shown that EGCG helps protect against several types of cancer by blocking the action of carcinogens. One study showed that women who consumed mushrooms and green tea have a 90 per cent lower incidence of breast cancer. EGCG in green tea is also very effective in increasing levels of friendly bacteria in the gut, and helping regulate and promote bowel health. Green tea also blocks the attachment of the bacteria associated with dental cavities, making it a great post-nosh drink!

The EGCG found in green tea can promote healthy and natural weight loss. The weight loss effects of supplementing your diet with green tea are not immediate, but they can be significant. Green tea can help you lose weight by increasing your metabolic rate and helping burn fat in the body while reducing the storage of fat. Green tea's calorie-burning properties lie in EGCG's ability to increase heat production (or thermogenesis) by affecting enzymes in the metabolic process and increasing the amount of calories burned throughout the day. *Now that's hot!* Although green tea does not produce immediate weight loss, green tea extract has been shown to stimulate fat oxidation and boost the metabolic rate without increasing the heart rate. And a faster metabolism means a slimmer you!

A randomized and controlled trial done at Oklahoma State University, in which thirty-five subjects with obesity consumed either four cups of green tea or two capsules of green tea extract a day over an eight-week period, found that green tea consumption significantly decreased both body weight and BMI (body mass index) versus the control group at eight weeks.

HOW TO USE: Adding green tea to your daily regime is a great idea for weight loss and to take advantage of all its fantastic health benefits. But bear in mind that it contains caffeine, so consuming it regularly in large amounts — or right before bed — is not necessarily recommended. The polyphenols in green tea are also active in the body, and may interfere with medications you may be taking, so you should consult a physician before prescribing yourself a strict diet of green tea. However, go ahead and drink up in moderation and enjoy reaping the wide range of health benefits EGCG has to offer.

Maca
Our favorite aphrodisiac from the chapter on sex can also help out in the hormone and weight-loss department. Maca is an adaptogen that helps to balance hormones naturally. It does this by nourishing, strengthening and balancing the endocrine system including your thyroid, pancreas and adrenals glands. Each of these play an important role in weight loss and while maca doesn't actually affect hormone levels, it does help to improve the communication between receptor cells. In order for the body to function optimally, hormonal communication must be kickin' seamlessly. A balanced thyroid keeps your metabolism burning, and balanced adrenals keep cortisol levels in check. As you'll learn in chapter 8, excess cortisol and insulin resistance are the main causes of excess belly fat. PLUS, maca contains Indol-3-carbinol (I-3-C), which helps to reduce the amount of bad, fat-storing estrogen that tends to sabotage weight-loss efforts. Wicked.

HOW TO USE: To banish the bulge with maca, you'll need 1500 to 3000 milligrams daily. For all the goods on other ways to use maca, check out chapter 4.

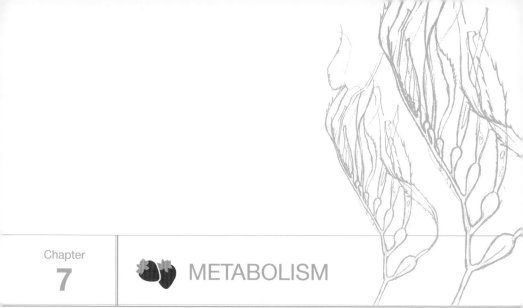

METABOLISM

I try and try but the scale doesn't budge! Sound all too familiar? Your thyroid is directly responsible for your metabolism. Period. It produces two hormones (T-3 and T-4) that control your body temperature and the rate at which your body uses and expends energy (carbs, fats and proteins). The thyroid also regulates your hormones and hormonal communication.

How your thyroid makes you fat (or skinny)
It's really quite simple: your thyroid drives your metabolism. When everything's in balance, it cruises along at a consistent speed. But when it gets out of whack — from things like poor nutrition or stress — your metabolism comes to a grinding halt worse than Friday afternoon traffic before a long weekend.

Since a picture speaks a thousand words, here a quick run through of how it all works:
- Your pituitary gland is an endocrine gland, about the size of a pea, that sits in the base of the brain. The pituitary gland helps control many body processes, one being thyroid gland function.
- Your hypothalamus is an area at the base of your brain that acts as a thermostat for your whole system. The hypothalamus signals your pituitary gland to make a hormone called thyroid-stimulating hormone (TSH).
- Your pituitary gland then releases TSH — the amount depends on how much T4 (thyroxine) and T3 (triiodothyronine) are in your blood.
- Your thyroid gland regulates its production of hormones based on the amount of TSH it receives.
- Although this process usually works well, the thyroid sometimes fails to produce enough hormones.

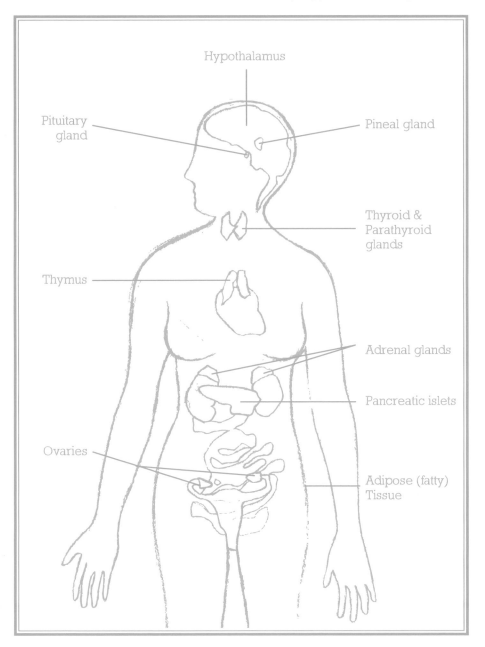

Hypothalamus

Pituitary gland

Pineal gland

Thyroid & Parathyroid glands

Thymus

Adrenal glands

Pancreatic islets

Ovaries

Adipose (fatty) Tissue

There are some nutrients that are must-haves and must-avoids when it comes to keep your thyroid performing at its peak:

Iodine
Even the slightest dip in your thyroid levels can send your metabolism to a crashing halt. In order for your thyroid to function optimally, it needs to absorb iodine from your blood, which enables it to manufacture and distribute hormones throughout your body. If adequate amounts of iodine aren't absorbed, your thyroid and metabolism become sluggish, and you can kiss precious fat-burning buh-bye.

Goitrogens
Goitrogens are naturally-occurring substances that can interfere with the function of the thyroid gland. If you suffer from a sluggish thyroid, it's best to avoid raw foods containing goitrogens. But many of these foods are necessary staples in the food connection to vibrant health, so don't cut them out altogether! Instead, I would suggest eating these foods cooked instead of raw, as cooking will destroy goitrogens (and remember, this is only necessary if you have a sluggish thyroid). These foods include:
- All soy products
- All raw cruciferous vegetables: broccoli, brussels sprouts, cabbage, cauliflower, kale, kohlrabi, mustard, rutabaga and turnips
- Millet
- Peanuts
- Radishes
- Spinach
- Strawberries
- Peaches

FOODS TO HELP SUPPORT THYROID FUNCTION

Kelp
Kelp is sea veggie that gives you the best of both worlds by satisfying your salt cravings while being low in sodium and packing a huge nutritional punch! Even though it's low in sodium, it tastes salty thanks to its rich complement of potassium, magnesium and other mineral salts. It contains over 70 proteins, growth hormones, vitamins, enzymes, trace elements and minerals, including iodine, potassium, magnesium, calcium and iron. Kelp is a rich source of iodine, which is critical for healthy thyroid function. It can help overcome iodine deficiencies, boost metabolism and, as a result, shed some unwanted pounds. In addition, kelp is extremely alkaline, which supports the body's pH balance and improves overall health. It also helps to boost energy levels and aids in digestion. This is key because undigested food particles become toxic, and fat binds onto toxins, making them harder to get rid of. And because your body craves nutrients, not calories, proper digestion is vital because it helps your body assimilate

nutrients, keeping you satisfied (and away from that bag of chips!).

HOW TO USE: The saltiness of kelp granules makes it a great salt substitute —
especially if you have high blood pressure or are trying to reduce your sodium
intake. You can use it in soups, sauces, dressings, salads and pastas, or to
season any dish that requires salt. Kelp can also be taken as a supplement in
tablet, capsule, liquid or powder form. You can also purchase kelp noodles, which
make a great noodle or pasta substitute! At only 12 calories per cup, it makes it a
stellar skinny substitution!

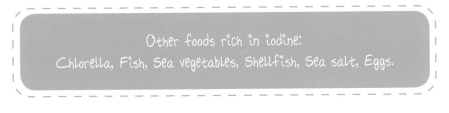

Other foods rich in iodine:
Chlorella, Fish, Sea vegetables, Shellfish, Sea salt, Eggs.

Other metabolism boosters
Sometimes our metabolism just needs a little pinch on the butt to give it a little
startle. Here are some foods that have thermogenic properties, which rev-up the
metabolism, burning more calories in the form of heat:

Cayenne pepper
This hot little number does a whole lot more than just spice up your meals
— cayenne is being increasingly seen as a miracle herb. Cayenne pepper, or
capsicum annum, is part of the nightshade family, and its cousins include bell
peppers and jalapenos. Apart from its use as a seasoning in spicy cooking
dishes, cayenne pepper is also used for medicinal purposes. The main ingredient
in cayenne is called *capsaicin*, which offers a plethora of important health benefits.

One of the most widely acclaimed health benefits of cayenne pepper is definitely
its role in weight loss. Yes, that's right! The capsaicin in these peppers can burn
extra calories in a similar way to exercise. A double-blind, placebo-controlled
study at the University of Maryland School of Medicine that studied the effects
of capsaicin on metabolism and weight loss in 40 men and 40 women over a
period of 12 weeks showed a decrease of abdominal fat in the capsinoid group
(which was not seen in the placebo group). Results also showed that capsinoid
indigestion was also associated with a significant increase in fat oxidation.

When taken regularly, cayenne pepper also helps facilitate weight loss by
increasing the body's metabolism. Cayenne is an active stimulant that increases
blood flow, which results in increased energy in the body. Increased energy
comes from the almost immediate strength the heart receives from the cayenne,
which means it has to pump less and leaves your body feeling energized.

However, it is necessary to clarify that cayenne will not magically cause weight loss, but rather acts as a catalyst for weight loss to occur. Regular use of cayenne pepper can be a fantastic tool to help increase metabolism and facilitate weight loss alongside a healthy balanced diet and an active lifestyle.

Cayenne pepper also has amazing benefits for the circulatory system, feeding the veins and arteries, reducing blood pressure, cleansing the arteries and helping rid the body of "bad" LDL cholesterol. Capsaicin also acts as a counter irritant, bringing up and carrying away blood toxins as well as reducing pain and inflammation. In fact, the heat from capsaicin increases our feel good endorphins — the same ones released after an orgasm or that give us that "runners high" after a great workout. When endorphins are released, they numb our pain receptors, reducing physical aches and pains.

Cayenne supports digestive function, stimulating peristalsis movement in our stomach and intestines and helping our bodies properly assimilate nutrients and eliminate efficiently. Believe it or not, it is also thought to heal tissues of the stomach when an ulcer is present, and its heat can do wonders to warm and soothe the body internally.

HOW TO USE: Add a small sprinkle to your meals and favourite dishes or use it a substitute for black pepper in cooking for some great "back of the throat" heat. And a little goes a long way! A dose as small as 1/16 of a teaspoon is enough to signal a physiological response on your body. Add some to your lemon water to jump-start your metabolism. I love adding a little cayenne to chocolate treats or spreads like hummus or guacamole for a little extra bite!

Yerba maté

Yerba maté is a South American herb and a member of the holly family. Yerba maté is rich in nutrients, including B-vitamins; vitamins A, C and E; and the minerals calcium, magnesium, iron, potassium and selenium, as well as powerful antioxidants. Researchers have indicated that yerba maté could be beneficial as a weight loss aid. They noticed a thermogenic effect in healthy individuals who took yerba maté, indicating a rise in the proportion of fat burned as energy.

HOW TO USE: Yerba maté is popularly consumed as a tea (it makes for a great coffee substitute) and can be made in a French press or espresso maker. It has also been extracted in supplement form used in many weight loss products.

BONUS: Other weight-loss tips

1. Add protein to your meals. Protein is a thermogenic which increases your metabolic rate 20-30% just by eating it. Add protein to each meal to increase satiety and boost metabolism. It also helps to stabilize blood sugar levels.

2. Add more calcium and vitamin D to your diet. Clinical studies published in the Journal of the American College of Nutrition show that for every 300 mg of calcium an adult consumes per day, is associated with a 2.5-3 kg lower body weight. But vitamin D appears to be even more important. Another study conducted by Ben-Gurion University indicates that those who increased both calcium and vitamin D intake lost nearly twice the weight than those who didn't.

3. Munch on low and negative calorie foods. Reach for foods like celery, lettuce, broccoli, and cabbage as the thermic effect of eating these foods pretty much wipe out the actual number of calories they contain.

Chapter 8 · MUFFIN TOPS

Sick of using wide belts and tunics to hide that extra mid-section bulge that hangs over the top of your jeans? Or, even worse, the dreaded horror of your hottie putting his arm around your "love handle" to find more than he bargained for? Fear no more, my friend. Off with the muffin top!

The two main contributors to belly fat are excess cortisol and insulin resistance. In this section, we're going to look at insulin resistance, but for more info on excess cortisol and tips on how to correct it, refer to Chapter 2 on stress — it's the same deal.

WHAT IS INSULIN RESISTANCE?

Insulin is a hormone responsible for moving sugar (glucose) from the bloodstream and storing it as glycogen within the muscles and liver so that it can be used as a source of energy. As sugars are absorbed into the bloodstream through diet and the digestion of carbohydrates, blood sugar levels rise. In order to lower blood sugar levels, the pancreas releases insulin, which moves sugar from the blood into the cells. The more refined the sugar, the greater the stress on the pancreas.

How excess insulin makes us fat

It's no secret that sugar causes weight problems and is linked to obesity, illness, diabetes, cardiovascular disease and mental health disorders. Although we need some sugar to function, too much can lead to big trouble. Once insulin is released, sugar is first used for immediate energy, particularly within your brain. Then it's stored in your muscles, then liver, and then whatever is left over is stored in your fat cells as, well, fat — especially in the tummy causing the dreaded muffin top. If that's not bad enough, the release of insulin not only causes excess sugars to be stored as fat, but the presence of insulin also shuts off our precious fat-burning hormones such as glucagon and human growth hormone.

Glucagon is a hormone that takes the fat out of storage and releases it so our bodies can burn it for energy. Human growth hormone (HGH) is responsible for growth, cell production and regeneration. It helps to build lean muscle, burn fat and has superior anti-aging benefits. We love HGH! But when your pancreas is pumping out the insulin in response to too much sugar, your body blocks the release of HGH and can't produce glucagons, two of the things that help us fight fat the most. So you end up storing extra fat while thwarting your body's attempts to burn it off at the same time. Oy.

The lowdown on sugar
If that's not enough reason to kick your sugar and refined-carb habits, get a load of these:

- Sugar feeds bacteria, yeast and candida, and contributes to both low blood sugar and high blood sugar. It also weakens the immune system and feeds diseases such as cancer.
- Over-consumption of sugar may also lead to constant fatigue (physical and mental), headaches, fast heartbeats, aches, muscular pains, shakes, loss of consciousness, paralysis, troubled vision and alcoholism.
- Hypoglycemia, which is low blood sugar brought on by too much insulin production, causes irritability, nervousness, moodiness, anxiety, fears and phobias, perception troubles, memory losses and concentration problems.

Insulin resistance
Remember, insulin is not the enemy. Insulin is required to move sugar from the blood into muscle and liver cells. But when your body is constantly circulating excess insulin, over time the cells get so used to it they start to ignore the fact that it's there. As they become less sensitive, the cell's uptake of glucose from the blood declines.

Think of it like online dating. The first time you try it you think, "Wow! This is great!" You literally have all these potential suitors just knocking on your inbox one after the other. Since each profile "virtually" appears to be the perfect catch, you eagerly and excitedly want to check all of them out, and you open each message as soon as it gets delivered, tingling with anticipation. After months of going on random dates, you either find that special person that rocks your world (congrats to you). Or, more likely, you want to throw your damn iPad out the freakin' window every time you hear that annoying "ping" reminding you of a new match that was delivered to your inbox. The appeal has obviously worn off. You ignore them and now you have all these unread messages flooding your inbox. Joy.

Insulin works the same way. Cells become less "eager and excited" by insulin's constant presence. Blood glucose levels remain high, since the cells couldn't be bothered to take in some of the insulin knocking at the door. In an attempt to manage the blood glucose levels, the pancreas creates even more insulin and starts to get flooded, like your inbox of unread messages. Your cells resist the insulin completely, hence the term *insulin resistance*. Once this happens, losing weight becomes a nightmare.

FOODS TO CHOP THE MUFFIN TOP

Yacon syrup

Who would have thought a sweetener could make you lose weight? But it can! In fact, this sweetener can actually lower your body mass index, reduce blood sugar levels and shrink your waist circumference. Hot damn! It's also rich in potassium and antioxidant vitamins A, C and E.

Yacon syrup is a sweetener extracted from the tuberous root of the yacon plant, native to Peru. Yacon root resembles a sweet potato, but has a much more fruity taste, although it is low in sugar and calories. And its blood-sugar-lowering properties make it not only safe but also beneficial for diabetics.

A 2009 study published in the *European Journal of Clinical Nutrition* indicated that yacon syrup demonstrated positive effects on obese, pre-menopausal women with insulin resistance. Over a 120-day, double-blind, placebo-controlled trial, obese and slightly dyslipidemic (containing an abnormal amount of fat and/or cholesterol in the blood) pre-menopausal women who were given yacon syrup every day had a significant decrease in body weight, waist circumference, body mass index and serum insulin levels. In addition, it helped increase satiety, helping them to feel fuller longer.

The rock star properties mainly come from yacon syrup's high concentration of fructooligosaccharide (FOS), which act as a pre-biotic fibre and stimulate colon health by improving intestinal flora. Because it's not digested, fibre is our fat loss BFF, as it gives us the full feeling without any calories. And since 30 to 50 per cent of this sweetener is comprised of FOS, that means up to half of it cannot be absorbed into the body, making it naturally low-cal and low-glycemic. FOS also helps with the absorption of calcium, another great weight-loss aid.

HOW TO USE: Yacon syrup has a thick, fruity, molasses-y taste and makes an awesome substitute for sugar or molasses in recipes, teas, cereals, oatmeal… or anywhere you can use a little sweetness in your life. However, because it has a pretty strong taste (and is slightly on the pricey side) you would want to use less than you normally would with regular sugar or sweeteners.

Cinnamon

Cinnamon is a great way to add a little sweetness to your life, helping to nix the muffin top sans the calories. This naturally sweet spice is found in the inner bark of the cinnamon tree. It has exquisite anti-microbial and antibacterial properties, and is also a great source of calcium, fibre, manganese, iron and antioxidants.

Not only can cinnamon replace sugar in your meals due to its innate sweetness, it can also lower the glycemic index of your food by stimulating your cells' insulin receptors, increasing their ability to absorb glucose and effectively lowering blood glucose levels. A study led by Pakistani researchers indicated that half a teaspoon (or one gram) of cinnamon a day can lower blood sugar levels in type 2 diabetics by 20 per cent. After the 40-day study period, not only were fasting glucose levels lowered, but so were triglycerides, "bad" LDL cholesterol and total cholesterol levels. Richard Anderson, who was part of this study, went on further and, in cooperation with the Beltsville Human Nutrition Research Center at the USDA, studied the effects of cinnamon in 22 obese subjects who were classified as pre-diabetic. He concluded that water-soluble antioxidants found in cinnamon improved antioxidant levels by 13 to 23 per cent, which correlates to a reduction in fasting glucose levels and aids in weight loss. Cinnamon is also known to increase the body's thermogenic properties, temporarily boosting metabolism. The water-soluble antioxidant also has anti-inflammatory properties.

Want to know what else? Cinnamon sticks are the perfect thing for getting rid of bad breath! Not only do they leave your breath feeling fresh and get rid of odor, but they're antibacterial. The most effective way to eliminate bad breath is to kill the sulfur-producing bacteria that is causing the odor. Besides the fresh taste cinnamon leaves in your mouth, it's also naturally calorie-free and sugar-free, as opposed to candied mints. A cinnamon stick is super easy to keep in your purse and carry on a date with you when you want to freshen up. Keep some pieces in a mint container and just pop one in your mouth! Plus, the sucking and chewing will stimulate saliva flow, which help to wash out the odor-causing bacteria.

HOW TO USE: Because cinnamon is naturally sweet sans the sugar, it makes a great sugar substitute. Sprinkle ground cinnamon on your favorite dishes, use it as a natural sweetener in your coffee or tea, or on breakfast cereals or on a baked sweet potato or squash. Try baking some apple slices sprinkled with cinnamon for a guilt-free treat.

Chia seeds

Cha-cha-cha chia! Yep, I'm talking about the same seeds that grow on that odd-looking, 80's retro chia pet plant. But lo and behold, it doesn't only grow on your countertop. Chia (*salvia hispanica*) is an actual plant native to Mexico and Central America. Its seeds are one of the world's highest plant-based sources of fibre (four times more fibre than flax!), making it an amazing weight loss aid and blood sugar stabilizer.

Chia seeds are a good source of omega 3 fatty acids (which also aid in weight loss) plus a plethora of antioxidants and other nutrients such as calcium and iron. Its high concentration of insoluble fibre soaks up fluids like a sponge. This increases levels of satiety, keeping you fuller longer. Fibre slows down the absorption of carbohydrates and improves the intake of sugar by cells and tissues. This helps balance blood sugar levels and wards off cravings. Fibre also lowers cholesterol levels, boosts heart health, pulls toxins from your body and improves digestive health. And as the toxins are eliminated, they take fat with them!

Chia seeds are also rich in protein, which delays hunger and has thermogenic properties, requiring more energy to be burned. Remember, your body craves nutrients, NOT calories! And because chia seeds are so nutritionally dense, your body won't be left craving more to be satisfied.

HOW TO USE: It's best to add the whole seed to something moist, as the high fibre content enables the tiny little seed to hold up to 20 times its weight in water! As such, it will start to plump up and absorb liquid. Your best options are adding it to a cereal, oatmeal or yogurt. You can also make a chocolate "tapioca-like" pudding by adding one tablespoon of the seed to a quarter cup of almond milk mixed with unrefined cocoa power. After a few hours in the fridge, the seeds will have pulled in most of the liquid, creating a pudding-like snack. YUM.

Bilberries
Bilberry is the euro-chic relative of the westernized blueberry. Closely resembling wild blueberries, bilberries are smaller in size but have a darker interior flesh due to their high-antioxidant anthocyanin pigments. In addition to their antioxidant, anti-inflammatory, skin-loving, belly-bloat-busting properties, bilberries have been used traditionally to balance blood sugar levels and even treat diabetes.

In a 2010 study published in the *Journal of Nutrition*, Japanese researchers tested the effects of bilberry extract on type 2 diabetic mice. They found the bilberry extract significantly reduced blood glucose concentrations and increased the uptake of insulin by activating a protein in fat tissue, muscle tissue and the liver. Their results suggest that bilberry extract is beneficial in the prevention and treatment of type 2 diabetes.

Bilberry is an extremely rich source of chromium, a mineral which helps maintain normal blood sugar and insulin levels and reduces carb cravings. Studies have shown that those who supplemented with chromium had the largest reduction in carb cravings. Bilberry leaves are particularly rich in tannins and myrtillin, a compound which also controls blood sugar levels.

HOW TO USE: Bilberries can often be found preserved as a jam, as frozen berries or in a liquid extract. The leaves are often used as a tea to treat blood sugar imbalances. Larger doses of 80 to 160 milligrams three times per day are recommended to treat diabetes.

Romaine lettuce

Romaine lettuce not only makes a great salad staple, but can actually help shrink your muffin top! Its secret ingredient? Chromium. Chromium is a mineral that helps to maintain normal blood sugar and insulin levels, and is key in carbohydrate and fat metabolism. Not only that, but it helps reduce sugar cravings!

Chromium plays a lead role in controlling blood sugar levels and is the active component in the body's glucose tolerance factor (GTF), which essentially helps to fulfill insulin's mission in life — to bring glucose to the cells to be used up for energy. Basically, what chromium does is lights a fire under your insulin receptors' ass, so instead of them resisting insulin, they actually increase their uptake, helping stabilize and lower blood sugar levels. This is especially key in the prevention and treatment of type 2 diabetes. Plus, it curbs weight gain and visceral fat (the harmful fat that hugs your organs).

And if you're the type that has a secret love affair with carbs and fats — 'specially when "emotional eating," chromium can kick those crazy cravings to the curb too! A study shown in the *Journal of Psychiatric Practice* indicated that when those who suffered from event-driven mood swings (i.e. atypically depressed) supplemented with chromium, there was a decrease in appetite and overeating, reduced carbohydrate cravings and fewer mood swings. So you can kiss that tub of ice cream buh-bye.

These crispy leafy greens are a great source of dietary fibre. Three cups of romaine contain 12 per cent of your daily recommended intake, also helping to slow down and stabilize blood sugar levels and supporting proper digestion, elimination and weight control. It is also high in vitamin A, C, K and folate, which are all essential vitamins and minerals for the body. Manganese is also an important trace mineral found abundantly in romaine lettuce. Like chromium, manganese also plays a role in maintaining healthy blood sugar levels in the body, and acts to prevent and/or treat type 2 diabetes.

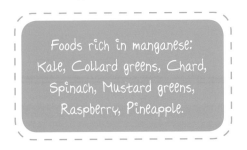

Foods rich in manganese:
Kale, Collard greens, Chard,
Spinach, Mustard greens,
Raspberry, Pineapple.

Although romaine lettuce is one of the richest sources of plant-based chromium, four cups only accounts for 26 per cent of your required daily intake. Combine with other some other sources of chromium, which include onions and ripe tomatoes as well as whole grains, oysters and potatoes.

For those who are insulin resistant, 200 to 400 milligrams of chromium is recommended per day, which may be best to take in supplement form.

HOW TO USE: Romaine not only makes for a great Caesar salad, but the crisp romaine leaves make a fun and super slimming substitution for taco shells, sandwich wrappers, dippers for hummus, guac or salsa and canapés. Try filling a romaine leaf with hummus, salsa, Kalamata olives and sprouts for satiating, fibre-rich snack.

> Foods high in chromium:
> Onion , Brewer's yeast, Sweet potato, Garlic, Broccoli, Green beans, Potatoes, Basil.

> TIP: For those who are insulin-resistant, 200 to 400 milligrams of chromium is recommended per day, which may be best to take in supplement form.

FOOD-BEAUTY CONNECTION

Discover the food secrets the beauty companies don't want you to know!

BEAUTY & ANTI-AGING

Girl, want the glow? Here's the first thing you can do for a radiant, flawless complexion. Walk into your bathroom. Grab your most expensive over-the-counter, anti-wrinkle cream and throw it out. Yes, I said throw it out. Now! In the garbage! These synthetic anti-aging creams may have a few "effective" compounds in there, but they can also be laced with chemical solvents that do more damage than good. And do you know what kind of damage? Wrinkle-causing ones! Yes, anti-wrinkle creams can actually cause wrinkles! The chemical ingredients that make up these expensive products can actually stress the skin. An allergic or anti-inflammatory response can occur, causing free-radical damage. The result: premature aging.

Beauty really does come from within. What you see on the outside is a direct reflection of what goes on inside you. I'm not just talking about the nutrients (or lack thereof) you put inside your body, but also what goes on in your thoughts — your mental state, your attitude towards yourself, your body image. And, as we've seen in the previous chapters, food does affect all of this. So to look glam out the outside, you need to start by feeling glam on the inside. Sure, you can use a good bronzer, but what happens when you're watching a rom-com with your sweetie and a tear trickles down your face, washing that sun-kissed glow away like a dirty river? Not feeling so hot then, are ya?

Why we age
Our body is made up of trillions of cells. The reason we age is because our cells accumulate free-radical damage over time. When a cell oxidizes, it loses an electron and free-radical damage occurs. Free-radical damage is caused by many factors, including metabolism, poor diet, environment, pollution, UV rays,

stress, allergies, pesticides, radiation and over-exertion. All of these things can cause the atoms or molecules that make up a cell to become unstable. This leads to oxidative cell damage, DNA damage, premature aging and diseases such as cancer and heart disease.

Here's an example of how this works. Let's say you have the full DVD box set of Glee. You go to play disc two and realize — it's missing! So you freak out a little, then decide that the next time you visit your sister you'll steal one of her discs to complete your set (after all, she's probably the one who took yours in the first place). The problem with this is that she is now left with an incomplete set. So she starts to freak out, becomes highly-reactive and sets out to take someone else's disc, causing a chain of events. The problem is someone is always left with an incomplete set and, in the process of all the shuffling around, the set gets damaged.

This is what happens to your cells. If an atom or molecule loses an electron, it becomes unstable. During this process, oxidative damage occurs and the cell begins to break down. So it starts to freak out, becomes highly-reactive, and begins the process of hunting down an electron from other cells in your body. A vicious chain reaction occurs causing widespread cellular disruption, oxidation, breakdown and damage.

The same holds true if you're stuck with an extra disc that doesn't fit into your box set. Let's say you later found your missing disc tucked away in another DVD case (oops!). So now you return your sister's copy, but she's already replaced hers by taking someone else's and now she's stuck with an uneven number. Free-radical damage occurs when there is an unpaired electron. The molecule will either scavenge your body trying to either steal an electron to complete its pair, or dump an extra it has no room for. Once a molecule either loses or gains an electron, the chemical structure changes and damage occurs. If free radicals go unchecked, they damage cells and can even alter DNA — mutating or deforming your genetic blueprint.

Antioxidants
Antioxidants prevent oxidation by neutralizing free radicals. They do this by taking up the space of the missing electron, making it complete. In the case of the missing DVD, it would be like ordering the one individual disc online, rather than stealing it from someone else. That way everyone has a complete set, no feathers get ruffled, no chain reactions occur and everyone's happy!

However, once these antioxidants give up one of their own electrons they become inactive, which is why we need to consistently add them to our diet. They are helpers. Instead of disrupting our own cells within our body (such as skin, muscles, heart, liver), antioxidants donate themselves, keeping our cells intact. How sweet!

These chain-breaking antioxidants include vitamin A (beta carotene), vitamin C (ascorbic acid), vitamin E, phytochemicals found in plant-based foods, ubiquinone, uric acid, and preventative-type enzymes such as superoxide dismutase, catalase and glutathione peroxidase. These work by destroying free radicals and making them "passive" so they don't react.

KEY NUTRIENTS FOR LOOKING YOUR BEST

Vitamin C (ascorbic acid)
Vitamin C firms and tones up the skin. It prevents free-radical damage, protects your skin cells and slows down the appearance of aging by preventing wrinkles. It's required for collagen production, as well as for the protection of collagen fibres that keep skin firm. Collagen is a protein molecule that makes up the dermis. This is what acts as the foundation of the skin and determines its firmness. The stronger the network of collagen fibres, the firmer the skin.

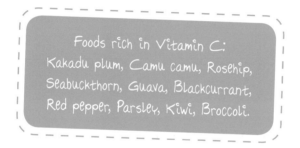

Foods rich in Vitamin C:
Kakadu plum, Camu camu, Rosehip, Seabuckthorn, Guava, Blackcurrant, Red pepper, Parsley, Kiwi, Broccoli.

Vitamin E
Vitamin E keeps moisture in the skin and protects the oils in the skin's moisture barrier from free-radical damage. It soothes dry skin and can minimize the appearance of wrinkles when applied topically. Vitamin E also reduces the effects of sun exposure on the skin and can help prevent skin cancer.

Foods high in vitamin E:
Sunflower seeds, Almonds, Walnuts, Mustard greens, Swiss chard, Spinach, Collard greens, Tomatoes, Turnip greens, Avocadoes, Mangos, Pine nuts.

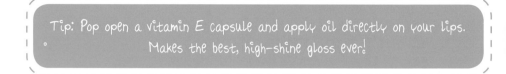

Vitamin A

Vitamin A helps normalize oil production in the skin and fights acne and inflammation. It also revitalizes the skin by increasing cell turnover and encouraging new skin cell growth. Eating real food sources of vitamin A or beta carotene (a pre-cursor to vitamin A) is the best way to ingest this nutrient. Too much vitamin A (in supplement form) can have negative health implications and increase your risk of hip fractures.

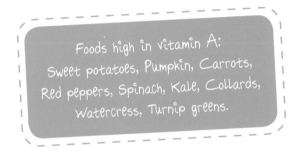

Foods high in vitamin A:
Sweet potatoes, Pumpkin, Carrots, Red peppers, Spinach, Kale, Collards, Watercress, Turnip greens.

Carotenoids

Carotenoids are strong antioxidants that protect against free-radical damage, provide anti-aging benefits, and enhance the immune system. There are roughly 50 different carotenoids. Here are a few:

Lycopene, the bright red carotenoid, acts as a natural sunscreen, protecting the skin from UV damage, which causes free radicals and results in wrinkles, dry skin and sun spots. Lycopene also helps build our skin-firming collagen.

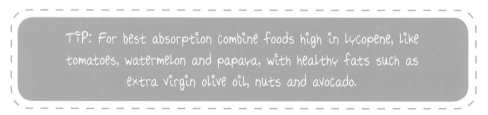

TIP: For best absorption combine foods high in lycopene, like tomatoes, watermelon and papaya, with healthy fats such as extra virgin olive oil, nuts and avocado.

Beta carotene, the most popular carotenoid, converts in the body to retinol, which is an active form of vitamin A. It has strong anti-aging benefits and protect against oxidative stress and UV damage. Beta carotene also enhances immune function and is known to help with male reproductive health. It provides the yellow-to-red pigments found in foods.

Lutien, another carotenoid, is excellent for eye health. Foods rich in lutien include spinach, chlorella and kale, so load up on those greens if you want to keep your eyes shining bright.

Polyphenolic antioxidants
Anthocyanins are powerful antioxidants that provide the deep red, purple and blue pigments found in plant-based foods, and are what give berries their claim to fame. They slow down the aging process — not only physically, but also mentally by keeping the brain sharp and preventing neurological decline. They also boast amazing anti-cancer properties and protect against diabetes.

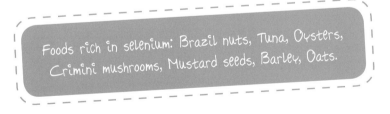

Foods high in anthocyanins: Purple corn, Chokeberries, Black raspberries, Wild blueberries, Red grapes, Cherries, Blackcurrants, Raspberries.

Resveratrol has anti-aging, anti-cancer and anti-inflammatory benefits, and can also help control blood-sugar levels. It is found in the skin of red grapes, and becomes most active during fermentation, making red wine the highest source. Wahoo!

Polyphenols are antioxidants with amazing health benefits. Red grapes, black currents, green tea and red wine are all great sources.

Selenium
Selenium aids in the production of the antioxidant enzyme glutathione, which repairs cell damage and slows down the skin's aging process. Selenium also supports the elasticity of our tissues and protects against sunburn and skin cancer.

Foods rich in selenium: Brazil nuts, Tuna, Oysters, Crimini mushrooms, Mustard seeds, Barley, Oats.

Zinc
Remember zinc, our super sex-drive-boosting nutrient? Zinc not only helps you feel good, but look good too! It's essential in the creation of new skin cells and aids in protein synthesis and collagen formation. It controls the production of oil in the skin and adds colour and brightness to the complexion. Got an acne problem? Acne is often a sign of zinc deficiency. So if you want clear, bright skin, get more zinc in your diet!

Copper

Copper is one of the most abundant minerals in our body and, along with zinc and manganese, is essential in the production of superoxide dismutase — the enzyme found in the skin that repairs all damage caused by free-radicals and produces skin-building cells. It also aids in the production of collagen and is what gives colour to hair, skin and eyes. A copper deficiency could cause premature graying, so you might want to swap your hair dye for some copper-rich foods.

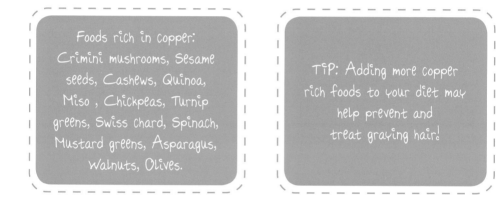

Foods rich in copper:
Crimini mushrooms, Sesame
seeds, Cashews, Quinoa,
Miso , Chickpeas, Turnip
greens, Swiss chard, Spinach,
Mustard greens, Asparagus,
Walnuts, Olives.

TIP: Adding more copper
rich foods to your diet may
help prevent and
treat graying hair!

Silica

Silica is a trace mineral essential for healthy skin. It strengthens connective tissues, tendons, cartilage, muscles, hair and nails. Silica improves your skin's elasticity and helps repair wounds. The best sources of silica are extracts derived from bamboo or horsetail. If horsetail's not your thing, try some of my other suggestions!

Foods rich in silica: Leeks, Cucumber skin,
Green beans, Chickpeas, Strawberries.

Omega-3 fatty acids

We covered omega-3s in detail in chapter 5, so you know how good they can be for boosting your mood. But omega-3s also help slow down the aging process and restore moisture to dry skin.

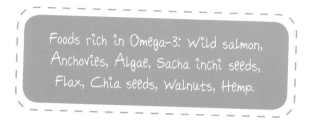

Foods rich in Omega-3: Wild salmon, Anchovies, Algae, Sacha inchi seeds, Flax, Chia seeds, Walnuts, Hemp.

FOODS THAT'LL HAVE YOU LOOKING SMOKIN' HAWT

Gogi berries

Goji berries (also known as wolfberries) are one of the most beautifying fruits around. They're like a makeover for your whole body — inside and out! Start adding this superfood to your diet and watch the transformation begin! Goji berries are among the highest antioxidant-containing foods and are thought to help fight heart disease, defend against cancer and diabetes, strengthen the immune system, improve vision, improve skin complexion and contain anti-aging properties. Their claim to fame is their high concentration of carotenoids, in particular beta carotene and zeaxanthin, both of which are essential for eye health and night vision. Beta carotene converts into antioxidant vitamin A, which helps treat acne. Gogi berries are also rich in polysaccharides. These polysaccharides, in combination with the gogi berry's exceptionally high source of antioxidant vitamin C, prevent against age-induced free-radical damage. One of the polysaccharides in particular appears to stimulate the secretion of HGH (human growth hormone) by the pituitary gland. HGH not only helps keep your skin young and firm, but it also increases lean muscle mass and aids in fat loss.

Goji berries' therapeutic applications include relieving fatigue, promoting visual health, protecting against diabetes, enhancing male sexual function and supporting a healthy life span. They contain 18 amino acids — including all the essential amino acids. As a rich protein source, goji berries are great for healthy looking hair! They also contain 21 trace minerals and are rich in B-vitamins and vitamin E. They also contain polysaccharides, which help strengthen the immune system. Goji berries have been traditionally regarded as a longevity and strength-building food — and no wonder!

HOW TO USE: Gogi berries are a tiny dried fruit with a tart taste. Toss them into oatmeal, cereals or muffin and cookie recipes. They can be re-hydrated in water and blended into a puree to be drizzled onto your favourite treat (try some over a sliced-up mango) or stirred into yogurt. They can also be added to boiling water and steeped into a tea.

Camu camu berries
The camu camu tree, grown in the rainforest of Peru, produces a powerful little fruit called the camu camu berry. Camu camu berries are one of the world's richest plant-based sources of antioxidant vitamin C, which helps with collagen formation. Collagen is the protein that gives your skin its structure, elasticity and tautness — in other words, youthfulness. Camu camu is also rich in antioxidants and flavonoids, both of which help prevent the free-radical damage that causes premature aging and disease. In addition, the vitamin C in camu camu is great for boosting the immune system and keeping you healthy and radiant inside and out!

HOW TO USE: Camu camu can be found in powder or supplement (capsule) form. The powder can be blended into smoothies or even applied topically. Because vitamin C is best used topically for the synthesis of collagen production in the skin, you can blend camu camu powder with coconut oil or extra virgin olive oil. Gently massage the mixture into your skin then wipe off with a damp cloth.

Olives & extra virgin olive oil
Olives aren't just for martinis! Olives (and extra virgin olive oil) are one of the healthiest fruits around — and one of the best-kept beauty secrets. Their high-antioxidant, antiviral, antibacterial, anti-inflammatory, anti-fungal properties treat a large number of diseases and ailments, including heart disease, several cancers (breast cancer, prostate cancer and colorectal cancer), candida, fungal infections, the flu virus and yeast infections. Olives can be used to lower cholesterol, protect the liver, guard against colitis, reduce inflammation, and improve the look of your hair and skin, giving you the glow!

Olives are a rich source of vitamins A and E, both of which protect the oils on the surface of your skin from free-radical damage. Olives also help strengthen connective tissues, improving skin tone and protecting against UV radiation. The rich phenol content protects skin against oxidization. By using extra virgin olive oil topically, you can prevent and treat aging skin. In addition, used topically, olive oil's antibacterial and anti-fungal properties can treat acne, eczema and psoriasis. It helps repair cells, protects against damage and soothes the skin, helping it renew and regenerate.

Extra virgin olive oil also helps with the absorption of calcium, contributing to bone health. The fats are made up primarily of monounsaturated fatty acids (heart-healthy because they raise good cholesterol) and cancer-fighting oleic acids, which moisturize and lubricate skin cells. It's naturally rich in squalane, which is a key ingredient in many store-bought skincare products. Squalane absorbs easily into the skin, keeping skin moist as well as restoring lost moisture.

Tip: Buying Olives

When choosing olives, it's best to choose dark purple or black olives due to their higher antioxidant properties and richer nutrient profile. Kalamata olives are my personal fave. It's the Greek in me! These olives contain the antioxidant anthocyanin, which is anti-aging, antibacterial, and anti-inflammatory, and can prevent and slow down the effects of cancer. However, do not buy those black, processed olives found in cans. Those have been chemically ripened and processed, and their nutrients destroyed.

Tip: Buying extra virgin olive oil

- Extra virgin olive oil (EVOO) is the highest quality olive oil and is made through an extraction process that does not alter or treat the oil in any way. When purchasing extra virgin olive oil, make sure it's in a dark glass bottle, as light, heat and oxygen destroy the nutrients and antioxidant properties and accelerate the oxidization process. Olive oil starts to degrade the moment it is squeezed from the olive, which is why it's essential the oil is stored in a dark bottle away from light.

- Use EVOO raw or cooked at extremely low temperatures. Drizzle it on food after the food has been prepared or use as a dressing. Heat destroys the phenols and antioxidant properties of the oil. EVOO has a low smoking point, around 250° F. Beyond that point the oil will smoke, oxidize and become rancid, causing further free-radical damage, which will cause, not prevent, premature aging!

- Virgin olive oil undergoes the same process as extra virgin olive oil but is made from olives harvested later in the year, giving it higher levels of acidity (between 0.8 per cent and two per cent, which distinguishes it from EVOO, which has an acidity of less than 0.8 per cent). Virgin olive oil has a higher smoking point than EVOO (around 350° F), which makes it better for cooking, but still keep it at a low temperature.

- If it's not extra virgin or virgin, do not buy it! The "olive oil" sold in clear glass bottles should not be used at all — ever! These are chemically treated, refined and devoid of nutrients and antioxidants. Oxygen attaches to the fats (oxidization) to produce hyperperoxides. Then the hyperperoxides break down and cause rancidity. Rancid oils cause free-radical damage in our body, which leads to disease and premature aging.

Note on cooking oils

Polyunsaturated fats are the worst oils to cook with. They are the most unstable and become rancid when exposed to light, heat and oxygen. These oils include all omega-3s and omega-6s such as hempseed oil, flax oil, safflower oil and corn oil. Most omega-6 vegetable oils are already rancid by the time you buy them. Coconut oil is the best oil to cook with at higher temperatures, followed by ghee or organic butter. Because of their saturated fat content, they are the most stable at high heats.

HOW TO USE:

- Add olives to salads, tomato sauces (olives and tomato sauce make a great antioxidant combo, especially to help against UV damage and protection), and other dishes to add a natural saltiness. When making a decadent chocolate dessert, blend in one black olive instead of the pinch of salt to bring out the richness and depth of the chocolate flavour. You won't even taste the olive, but it does an amazing job of bringing out the richness of the chocolate. Olives are also great blended in chocolate smoothies.
- Drizzle extra virgin olive oil onto already-cooked dishes and use in salad dressings.
- Use extra virgin olive oil topically as a moisturizer. Your skin will absorb the oil and it won't leave you greasy.
- Smooth EVOO onto lips as a natural moisturizer and lip gloss.
- Use EVOO as a facial moisturizer before bed, especially around the eye area.
- Add the oil to a warm bath and soak in it for supple skin.
- Soak your fingernails in oil to soften cuticle and strengthen nails. Adding fresh, minced garlic increases the anti-fungal properties.
- Mix EVOO with sea salt and rub onto skin as an exfoliant to remove dead skin cells.

Coconut oil

If you want the glow, you have to get fat. The healthy kind of fat found in foods like coconut oil, that is! Coconut oil is a great way to get those beauty-boosting essential fats without the extra calories that will lead to the wrong kind of fat. By weight, coconut oil has fewer calories than any other fat source. Although it's a saturated fat, the medium chain fatty acids make it easily absorbable by the small intestine (not requiring the full digestive process). This means it provides increased energy faster than any other fat. Coconut oil has immune-boosting properties and is antiviral, anti-microbial, and anti-fungal. It is especially beneficial to those who suffer from candida or fungal infections, which can lead to acne and skin irritations. So by adding more of this to your diet, you may begin to see your face clear.

Due to the fatty-acid profile, coconut oil is also great for topical use as a moisturizer. It can smooth and clear skin and may help reduce the signs of stretch marks. Because it's a saturated fat, it can help firm-up saggy skin. Saturated fats are required to strengthen cell walls, and plant-based sources are the healthiest. And, contrary to popular belief, research shows that coconut oil can also help lower cholesterol levels. It's also great for diabetics and helps normalize blood sugar levels. Whether it's eaten through food or used topically as a moisturizer, it does wonders for improving skin… making it totally succulent!

HOW TO USE: Coconut oil is a stable fat and has a high smoking point, making it great for cooking! Use coconut oil when sautéing, roasting or frying for a healthier alternative to other oils. It's also great added to smoothies, improving flavour and silkiness, as well as added to many desserts. Just replace the oil or butter with coconut oil. As a daily moisturizer, rub the oil onto the face and body for a healthy glow. I keep a small lip-balm sized container in my purse for instant, smoochable, delicious lips! It also makes a great eye-makeup remover!

The oil isn't the only nutritious part of the coconut, either. Coconut flour can replace regular flour in baked goods, coconut kefir makes a great probiotic and digestive tonic, coconut milk makes a great dairy alternative due to its rich and creamy consistency, and coconut water is nature's best sport energy drink. Coconut water is an exceptional source of electrolytes, which is great for marathon runners, those who do intensive sports and training, or for those who've had a little too much alcohol to drink!

Aloe
Aloe is a great plant to have around the house or in the garden — it's a medical powerhouse in a pot! The aloe plant is highly regarded for its anti-inflammatory and healing properties. It's especially beneficial in the treatment of skin conditions such as psoriasis, eczema, rosacea and herpes and can be used to quickly heal wounds, burns and frostbite if applied topically. Aloe can speed up the healing of bad burns by nearly nine days. The anti-inflammatory properties may be partially attributed to the plant's high concentration of methylsulfonylmethane (MSM). MSM is a natural sulphur compound that helps alleviate arthritic joint pain, inflammation, joint flexibility and strength. This also makes aloe gel great for muscle recovery after a workout. However, MSM is only found in outdoor plants fed by rainwater or sulfur-rich water. Ingesting aloe can also decreases the number and size of papillomas and reduces the incidence of tumors by more than 90 per cent in the liver, spleen and bone marrow.

Aloe is rich in polysaccharides, which also have anti-inflammatory properties and aid in the growth of new tissue. Polysaccharides have superior intestinal health benefits (such as improving digestion and reducing risk of colon cancer) and help your body absorb precious nutrients, keeping your health and glowing complexion in check. Since aloe is more absorbable than vitamin E, it makes a phenomenal emollient that soothes and softens dry skin.

HOW TO USE: Scoop out the gel from the inside of the aloe leaf to use topically as a skin treatment, gently massaging into skin. Or you can blend the gel into your favourite smoothie for additional anti-inflammatory properties, to aid in digestion, to help your body absorb nutrients and for overall health benefits.

Raw Honey

Need a little sweetness in your life? Try some raw honey to satisfy those sugar cravings while helping your body look and feel amazing! Raw honey is one of nature's most wondrous promoters of general health. This pure source offers so many health benefits that it is truly one of the world's food treasures. Raw honey is the only absolutely unprocessed honey, as it is unheated, unpasteurized and 100 per cent pure. Its health benefits come mainly from its abundance of naturally-occurring nutrients. Raw honey is nutritionally superior to all others forms of honey, as it contains loads of vitamins, minerals, amino acids and over 5,000 live enzymes. So it's not surprising that honey in its raw form acts as a powerful immune booster in the body. It is these powers that help your body fight off illness and disease and can give your digestive system a real kick-start.

Unlike most of the honey found in supermarkets, which has been pasteurized (heated) and filtered to look more appealing to the consumer (not to mention easier to spread), raw honey is in its pure form. The heating undergone by most commercial honey causes a destruction of many of the enzymes and yeasts that benefit the body. The bottom line: raw honey is much more nutritious than your average grocery version that has undergone any of these treatments.

Raw honey has antiseptic, antibiotic and antibacterial properties, and it is for these reasons it has been used for healing wounds, cuts and burns for centuries. These properties allow honey to inhibit bacterial growth and infection, as well as minimize pain and inflammation while promoting the body's natural healing processes. The *Journal of the Royal Society of Medicine* states that honey is a simple, convenient and effective topical remedy for infected non-healing wounds due to its antibacterial properties in vitro. The journal also notes that honey has been successfully used in the healing of chronic topical ulcers.

Research recently published in the *Journal of the Federation of American Societies for Experimental Biology* shows for the first time how honey kills bacteria. The research shows that bees make a protein added to the honey which can be used to treat burns and skin infections and could one day help combat antibiotic-resistant infections. Now, that's what you call superfood power!

HOW TO USE: On a day-to-day basis, these healing properties can also help facilitate the healing of blemishes and zits on skin. Just dollop some raw honey directly on your zit and watch it vanish. Honey is believed to have an overall positive effect on keeping skin healthy and vibrant. You may or may not already know that honey is an age-old beauty product that can help keep you looking youthful and beautiful. A spoonful daily in your tea is all you need to reap these amazing benefits! And a quick beauty tip — applying raw honey topically provides nutrients and draws moisture to the surface of the skin. Rub some on your face and lips, then wash off for a healthy and kissable glow. But keep in mind — it is sticky!

HOMEMADE BEAUTY PRODUCTS

Skin exfoliator	Ingredients • Strawberry — helps exfoliate skin • Oats — helps exfoliate skin • Camu camu powder — helps exfoliate skin • Raw honey — helps bring moisture to the surface of the skin In a bowl, mash up ½ cup strawberries, mix in ½ cup oats, add 1 tbsp camu camu powder and 1 tbsp raw honey. Massage onto face and skin. Rinse off with luke warm water.
Anti-aging moisturizer	Face • Extra virgin olive oil — This is your best bet! And no, it's not greasy. It will absorb into your skin keeping it soft and supple. Bonus: add a drop of sea buckthorn oil for added anti-aging benefits. • Almond Oil — Rich in skin softening vitamin E and will protect your skin from environmental pollutants. • Coconut oil — Works great but doesn't penetrate deep into the skin as well as extra-virgin olive oil does. Body • Coconut oil • Sea buckthorn — Has amazing anti-aging and skin rejuvenating benefits. It's rich in antioxidants and essential fatty acids. It treats skin conditions, acne, wrinkles, and wounds and has amazing skin restorative properties. Heat coconut oil, melting it into liquid form. Add a couple drops of sea buckthorn oil to ½ cup of coconut oil and mix well. Let oil solidify at room temperature and use as a restorative and rejuvenating body lotion.

Face mask	Ingredients • Buttermilk — Contains alpha-hydroxyacid (AHA) which rejuvenates skin and is often used in professional peels. • Avocado — The high fat-content and antioxidants vitamins A and E soften the skin. • Banana — Potassium revitalizes the skin. • Kiwi — High in antioxidants, vitamin C and antioxidant vitamin E Blend buttermilk, avocado, banana and kiwi in blender, rub onto skin and let it sit for 20 minutes. Then wash off with luke warm water.
Toner	Ingredients • Cucumber juice — Skin contains collagen-strengthening silica • Lavender oil — Rich in tannins to firm and tighten the skin Juice one cucumber with skin and add a couple of drops of lavender oil. Apply to a cleansing pad and gently apply to face in a circular motion. Or, you may pour into a spray bottle and use it as a spritzer to rehydrate skin.
Lip balm	Mix 4 parts coconut oil with 4 parts extra virgin olive oil and 1 part raw honey. Keep in a small container and apply to lip for an uber-moisturizing lip treatment.
Lip gloss	Pop open a vitamin E capsule and spread the oil directly on lips. Makes the best lip gloss ever! So shiny! You may even add cinnamon or peppermint oil to the mix if you want to increase their fullness, giving them a poutier, sexy look.
Body moisturizer	Ingredients • Apricot Oil — High in antioxidant vitamins A and C, and because it's applied topically, it will aid in collagen production. It's also easily-absorbed in your skin and doesn't have a strong scent (like olive oil). After all, I don't think you want to walk around smelling like a Greek salad. Plus, it's relatively inexpensive compared to other oils. • Almond oil — Also amazing, just a little more pricy! The best way to use it is to keep it in your shower, and as soon as you're done bathing, saturate your body with it. When your skin is moist, it yields the greatest absorption. You may also add your own natural fragrance using essential oils, such as lavender, lemon balm, angelica, cinnamon, citrus, or whatever your heart, and nose, fancies. Grapefruit will uplift and refresh you, while adding lavender can help relax you after a long day.

Cellulite treatment	Ingredients • Coffee — Caffeine temporarily reduces the appearance of cellulite by pumping up the area so the dimples aren't so noticeable. It helps to tighten skin, tightens blood vessels and reduces inflammation. • Coconut oil While there is no food, lotion, cream or chemical that will banish cellulite forever, there are some temporary fixes that can help reduce the cottage cheese effect that sits under your butt (or wherever it may be!) Mix ¼ cup of coffee granules with ¼ cup of coconut oil. Massage well onto skin and let sit for 15–20 minutes then wash off.
Acne zapper	Just dollop raw honey directly on your zit to zap it in no time!
Age-spot remover	Ingredients • Juice of a lemon OR • Licorice oil Apply directly to dark patches of skin or age spots and it will help the colour fade. Licorice oil/extract works great for rosacea as well.
Teeth whitener	Ingredients • Strawberries • Non-aluminum baking soda Mash up strawberries in a bowl then stir in some non-aluminum baking soda. Dip your toothbrush into the mixture and brush away all those stubborn stains. It will have your teeth looking pearly white!
Breath freshener	Ingredient • Cinnamon — Anti-bacterial so not only will it immediately freshen breath, but will kill odor-causing bacteria. Nix those candied mints for cinnamon sticks! Break a small piece of cinnamon stick and suck on it like a mint or mix 1 tbps ground cinnamon with water and gargle like mouthwash.

FOOD-HEALTH CONNECTION

Feel amazing every day with foods to boost immunity, improve digestion and beat the monthly PMS woes!

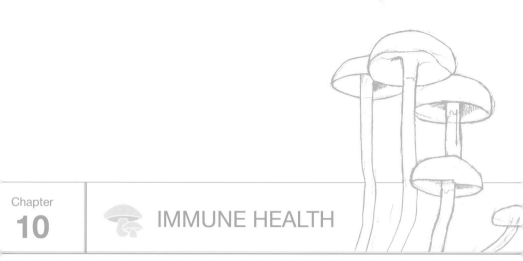

🍄 IMMUNE HEALTH

Our body has a pretty tough gig. We stay up too late, push too hard at work, don't always get the right foods in our diet and sometimes bitch at it for not looking as hot as we'd like in certain pairs of jeans. We need to take a moment and give it some love. We quite often take for granted how hard our body is working for us every second of the day. We are constantly being exposed to foreign organisms such as bacteria, viruses, parasites, fungi and microbes, and our bodies' defense systems are constantly kicking some serious microorganism ass. Take your saliva for example. It's not just for the joy of eating, digesting food or heavy duty smooching. It's actually part of your first line of defense for keeping pathogens out of your body. A healthy body and immune system is geared up to keep those harmful invaders away! However, if our defense mechanisms are compromised, we might be in for some trouble. Health issues arise when the immune system is unable to stop a disease in its initial stage.

HERE'S A LOOK AT HOW HARD YOUR BODY IS WORKING FOR YOU

First Line of Defense
Pathogens, like viruses, bacteria or microorganisms, first have to get into your body to do their damage. Your body comes equipped with plenty of barriers to keep the bad guys out — including your skin, mucus, saliva, tears and vaginal fluids. Keeping these barriers strong and healthy is an important first step in achieving a good immune health. Remember, your body is a temple — make it a fortress!

Second Line of Defense
This is the defense system that kicks in once a pathogen slips through those outer barriers and enters the body. If the first line fails, your body has a whole host of

other defenses just waiting in the wings.

As soon as a pathogen enters the body, an inflammatory response occurs. It's a protective measure to prevent the spread of injury and initiate healing. There are two kinds of inflammation: acute and chronic.

- Acute inflammation is short-term and typically the result of an injury. Our body sends neutrophils to deal with acute inflammation. They are cells that destroy pathogens at the acute phase of injury.
- Chronic inflammation is when the inflammation lasts longer than a couple of weeks. This stresses the immune system and could lead to disease if left untreated. This is when you need your macrophage cells, which not only destroy pathogens, but also present them to lymphocytes, which are cells that support the immune system.

Other invader-kicking members of the second line of defense are:
- Natural killer (NK) cells, which, ironically, "naturally kill" and destroy viruses and malignant cells. Yep — they're bad-ass like that.
- Fever. Yes it's true. Fever is another important defense mechanism, because the body promotes healing by increasing the metabolic temperature.

> **NOTE:** Foods can also be considered pathogens. If we ingest harmful substances or foods that our bodies are sensitive to, an inflammatory response can occur. Chronic inflammation can lead to a host of health problems and diseases, so pay close attention to how what you eat affects your body.

Third Line of Defense
If the pathogens make it this far, your immune system kicks into full throttle to get those invaders out of your body and eliminate the threat. In the second line of defense, the macrophage cells present the pathogens to lymphocytes, which are like the Godfather of defensive cells.

There are two types of these lymphocytes, and they tag-team to give you the best protection possible.
- T-cells are created in the thymus gland and destroy pathogens.
- B-cells are created in bone marrow and are responsible for antibody production.

For example, let's say you've been hit with this crazy flu. It's obviously crossed your first line of defense because it's now in your body and has created an inflammatory response. You're all mucus-y and fevered-up. So the second line, bad-boy macrophage cells attack the invader and present them to the third line lymphocyte cells. Here, the T-cells will work hard to destroy the flu bug and the B-cells will create specific antibodies against it. Go team.

The antibodies/immunoglobulins (Ig) created by the B-cells are proteins that fight against particular antigens, such as this stomach flu. If it's the first time you've been hit with this particular strain of stomach flu, the B-cells will create a specific antibody against it. Not only that, but these suckers are SO smart that once created, they will store them for future use so they will never have to create them again! So, if you get hit with the same virus again, the B-cells will evaluate and pull the appropriate fix from the file. Bet you didn't know your body was so smart, did ya? Brilliant.

KEY NUTRIENTS THAT BOOST YOUR IMMUNE SYSTEM

Vitamin D
Who doesn't love that sun-kissed glow? Even just the thought of it can make you feel healthier already! Well look no further. If you want to keep your immune system ready and raring to go at a moment's notice — give it a little sunshine! Studies show that people with low blood levels of vitamin D have significantly greater incidences of the cold or flu. Even more research suggests vitamin D can be just as effective (if not more effective) than obtaining the flu shot (not to mention that hitting the beach is way more fun). Adequate levels of vitamin D in the blood stream are essential in order for your body to activate its immune response and defend against invading, disease-causing microbes. Essentially, vitamin D is required to turn on an antimicrobial protein that fights against foreign invaders. Not only does it activate your immune system, it also prevents against inflammation brought on by the flu.

> TIP: The rule of thumb for Vitamin D is that you generally need 35 IU per pound of body weight.

The best way for your body to get vitamin D is through direct sunlight, which contains UVB rays. UVB helps your body manufacture its own vitamin D in the perfect amount by converting cholesterol in the skin to D3. However, if, like me, you live in the northern hemisphere and relish in the entire five minutes of sunshine you may get during the winter months, bundled in your parka and Uggs, it just won't cut it. Especially if that trip to Cabo just isn't on the radar this year, it's important to get your vitamin D through other means.

Vitamin D can be found in some fish oils, milk and dairy products, as well as egg yolks. However, vitamin D from food sources doesn't supply us with adequate amounts, which is why it's best to take a supplement during winter months. Although government guidelines hover around 200 IU per day, research suggests at least 2000 IU per day is necessary to ensure normal blood levels.

Antioxidant vitamins A, C and E

I know, I know — I've already gone on and on about how amazing antioxidants are for reducing stress and making you look and feel fab. But I can't help myself — they are just that awesome. Not only will they make you look and feel good, they'll keep your immune system strong and healthy by protecting it from the harmful effects of free-radical damage, which leads to disease. The following vitamins each have their own unique function:

Vitamin C is a powerful antioxidant that not only helps get rid of a cold or flu, but is essential to preventing it in the first place. Vitamin C increases the production of antibodies and white blood cells, which are key in fighting against infection. In particular, it increases levels of the antibody interferon, which coats cell walls and prevents the entry of viruses.

Since your body does not manufacture or store vitamin C, it's essential you add it to your daily routine. Fruits and vegetables are excellent sources. Camu camu berries are one of the world's highest plant-based sources of vitamin C (they can also be found in supplement form). Other excellent sources include goji berries, red bell peppers, strawberries, broccoli, Brussels sprouts, kiwi, lychees and parsley. And believe it or not, these ALL trump oranges in the amount of vitamin C they contain.

> Tip: Next time you're feeling run down, swap out your O.J. for a Vegatini (see page 131). It has over 60 times the amount of vitamin C, amongst other immune-boosting and anti-inflammatory nutrients.

Vitamin E is essential for healthy immune function. It is required for the production of immunoglobulins, the immune cell antibodies that destroy all those pathogens that try to do us harm. They're like your own personal bodyguard, standing by to protect you. And who said chivalry was dead? So give 'em some vitamin E love, and they'll love you back!

Beta carotene, which your body converts into vitamin A, also enhances the functioning of your immune system. It works by increasing the number of immune-boosting cells, including natural killer cells, required for normal T-cell metabolism and for the production of antibodies, which prevents entry of pathogens. Keep building that fortress babes.

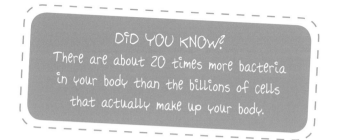

Probiotics

Probiotics literally mean "for life." Probiotics are live bacteria culture, and yes, you're supposed to eat them. Probiotics are live microorganisms classified as good bacteria that help fight off all the bad bacteria (foreign, disease-causing microorganisms). Eighty per cent of our immune system resides in the gut, and there are roughly 20 times more bacteria in your body than the actual billions of cells that make up your body! In order to keep our immune system strong we need to keep our intestinal system healthy with probiotics. They help improve immune function by increasing the number of T-lymphocytes (the virus-fighting white blood cells we call T-cells) and natural killer cells. Basically, they boost the immune system by increasing white blood cell count and by giving you more ass-kicking friends. Who can't use more of those? They prevent the over-growth of yeast, mold, fungal colonies, and other not-so-cool microorganisms, which are the precursors to diseases such as cancer and heart disease. They also treat yeast infections, vaginal infections and candida. When was the last time your BFF did that for you? Thought so.

Probiotics also improve digestion and help your body assimilate the precious vitamins and nutrients within your food. After all, you are not only what you eat, but what you assimilate! You could be eating extremely well, but if you don't have a good digestive system you could be missing out on all the good stuff.

Probiotics are naturally found in fermented foods such as miso, coconut kefir, yogurt, sauerkraut, kimchi, kombucha and fermented soy sauce. So make friends with bacteria — the good kind — and watch your immune and digestive systems flourish!

TIP: If you are taking a daily probiotic supplement, it's best to alternate between brands. Since different brands typically carry different strands of active bacteria culture, it's best to switch it up and confuse the bad bacteria in your system!

Beta glucans

Beta glucans are polysaccharides that have the ability to activate the immune system and prevent infections. They modulate white blood cells and keep them in a highly-prepared state so they are ready to attack should there be any threat to our immune system. Think of it like this: your local radio station announces that your fave band is doing a secret show somewhere in the city tonight, but you have to keep listening for clues. The radio DJ (aka the beta glucan) is making sure you (aka your white blood cells) are in a high state of excitement, constantly checking Facebook and Twitter and listening to the radio to find the clue to where the concert (the immune threat) will be. Once you find it, bam! You're all over that sucker. You go into party mode, and your white blood cells go into attack mode. What's also great about beta glucans is that while they activate the immune system, they don't cause over-stimulation, which can lead to auto-immune disease.

Beta glucans can be found in baker's yeast, the bran in grains such as oats and barley, as well as mushrooms, especially the shiitake, maitake and oyster varieties.

FOODS THAT BOOST YOUR IMMUNE SYSTEM

Mushrooms: reishi, shiitake, maitake, Agaricus blazei Murill, button

Who knew that those delicious pizza-toppers could boost your immune system and prevent diseases such as cancer? All mushrooms are rich in beta glucans. Beta glucans are polysaccharides and are among the strongest immune-boosting compounds around. They have strong anti-tumor properties and also activate the immune system and regulate disease-fighting white blood cells so that they are ready to attack against whatever comes its way. It's kind of like a military boot-camp for immune cells.

Not only do mushrooms activate the immune system, they are also rich in minerals, vitamins, polyphenols and sterols that also keep our immune system healthy and strong. Mushrooms are also one of the few foods that contain vitamin D. (However, because the amount of vitamin D in mushrooms is small in comparison to the daily-required intake, it's still best to supplement.)

Here are some of the top mushrooms containing medicinal (not to be confused with magical!) properties.

Agaricus blazei Murill	Agaricus blazei Murill (ABM) is native to Brazil, although widely cultivated in Japan, and is known as the "Mushroom of God." And rightly so! It contains the highest concentration of beta glucans compared to all other 'shrooms. ABM is also higher in protein, which helps support the immune response and stimulates macrophage activity.
Shiitake	Shiitake mushrooms contain a type of beta glucan called lentinan, which stimulates the production of white blood cells, has reported anti-cancer benefits, increases the quality of life of cancer patients and reduces the rate of cancer re-occurrence. These mushrooms are also very heart-healthy, as they lower cholesterol and can prevent heart disease.
Maitake	Maitake mushrooms have immune-boosting and cancer-fighting abilities, and studies show they can block tumor formation in mice.
Reishi	Reishi mushrooms increase the production of interleukins, which are cytokines that regulate the immune response and inflammatory reactions and inhibit tumor formation. They also contain strong anti-inflammatory, antioxidant, antibacterial and antiviral properties. Reishi mushrooms increase interferon production, which blocks viruses from spreading. They also protect against radiation.
White button	Researchers at Tufts University have concluded that white button mushrooms boost the immune system by increasing the production of proteins that fight disease-causing pathogens. They also increase the maturation of dendritic cells, which produce T-cells and fight against microbial invasion and tumor development.

HOW TO USE: Mushrooms seem to make everything taste better! Add them to pizza, pastas, sauces, salads soups or make a Mo'shroom Gravy for your Garlic Mash (recipe on page 150). You can purchase them fresh or dried. You can rehydrate the dried mushrooms by soaking in water and using the soaking water in sauces or as a soup stock.

Chlorella

If you want to save that next "sick" day for a "way-too-sunny-to-go-work" day, chlorella is a MUST in your nutrition arsenal. Chlorella keeps your immune system strong by keeping pathogens in check and fending off illness.

The two main constitutes of chlorella are chlorophyll and the Chlorella Growth Factor (CGF). Chlorophyll boosts immune function, reduces inflammation, helps eliminate toxins and promotes alkalinity. The more alkaline your body, the healthier and vibrant you will be. And when it comes to chlorophyll, chlorella is the richest source in the world!

The Chlorella Growth Factor (CGF), is literally a phenomenon. This jacked-up superfood increases tissue-building and repair (helping you look and feel fab), multiplies the 'good' active bacterial culture in your intestines (improving digestion, assimilation of nutrients and health) and supercharges white blood cell activity – all boosting your immune system, health and vitality. The CGF is made up of nucleic acids (RNA/DNA), in addition to proteins, peptides, polysaccharides, beta glucans, sulfur and manganese, which are found in the nucleus of the cell; all of which contribute to immune health. Therefore the higher the CGF, the better it is.

The polysaccharides, including beta glucans, found in the nucleus help activate the immune system and keeps it ready to attack. They help to increase macrophage activity, which are those bad-ass cells that destroy pathogens once they have entered our body. Then once the ass-kicking is done and the foreign invader is destroyed, macrophage will then carry small particles of the pathogen and present them to lymphocytes – in particular, T-cells, for final clean-up. And because of that, it's a good thing chlorella helps to activate and increase the production of T-cells and B-cells as well! T-cells mature in the thymus and destroy intercellular pathogens. B-cells matures in bone marrow and are responsible for antibody production (those plasma proteins that fight particular antigens, like, food allergies).

Chlorella is not only rich in antioxidants A, C and E, which prevent illness, but also protects against free-radical damage and boosts the immune system. It also activates our body's own, in-house, queen of antioxidants, superoxide dismutase (SOD) and glutathione peroxidase. These two powerhouses are produced within our body and are essential in fighting off free-radical damage and disease.

In addition, studies have confirmed that chlorella can provide critical benefits for the health of individuals with suppressed immune systems, especially when under extreme stress. The biggest benefit was shown in those who had undergone chemotherapy treatment. Chlorella demonstrated significant results in improving and strengthening the immune system.

HOW TO USE
For details on how to add chlorella to your life, take a look back at page 13.

Aphanizomenon flos-aquae (AFA)
Can algae help you cut down on sick days? Yep. Aphanizomenon flos-aquae (AFA) is a blue-green fresh water algae that's been around for, well, forever. It's

one of the most primitive life forms on Earth, and among the most nutrient-dense foods around. AFA embodies a plethora of vitamins (including B-vitamins and antioxidants A, C and E), minerals, trace minerals, phytonutrients, amino acids and essential fatty acids. It also has antiviral, antibacterial, anti-inflammatory, antioxidant and anti-cancer properties. Start adding this tiny superstar to your diet and you can start taking those sick days to go shopping! Just don't tell your boss I said that…

One of the key components to AFA's immune-boosting effect is attributable to phycocyanin. Phycocyanin is what gives AFA its blue pigment and constitutes up to 15 per cent of the alga's dry weight. Whereas the green pigment rejuvenates and strengthens blood through its rich chlorophyll content, the blue pigment strengthens immune function. Phycocyanin's antioxidant properties allow it to act as a free-radical scavenger, preventing disease, inhibiting inflammation and revving up stem cell production. Not only that, but the blue pigment is also a COX-2 inhibitor. The COX-2 enzyme is highly dominant in many breast cancer cells. Hence it's suggested that phycocyanin can result in reduced tumor growth.

A study conducted by McGill University researchers concluded that human consumption of AFA leads to rapid changes in immune cell trafficking. Just two hours after consuming one and a half grams of AFA, 40 per cent of the immune system's natural killer cells migrated from the blood stream to the tissues to work their magic. In addition, it resulted in increased blood cell counts of T-cells and B-cells, as well as monocyte subsets. An additional study showed that chickens that were fed blue-green algae had greater anti-tumor cell activity compared to those that went without. This suggests an increase in natural killer cell activity.

AFA is also rich in carotenoid antioxidants, including beta carotene, lycopene and lutein, which help prevent disease and reduce inflammation. It's also an excellent source of EPA and DHA (omega 3 derivatives), which help reduce inflammation, stabilize and strengthen cell membranes, speed up healing and assist in the production of pathogen-fighting antibodies and bacteria-eating white blood cells. Seriously, this blue piece of goo is packed with so many nutrients you'll be wondering where it's been all your life.

AFA's rich mineral profile includes iron, which is required for the production of antibodies and immune response, as well as zinc, which increases natural killer cells activity, increases macrophages activity and assists in the reproduction of DNA (and not just because it also boosts your libido!). It also helps detoxify the body, eliminate heavy metals and balance blood sugar levels.

If all this isn't enough reason, check this out. AFA is one of the highest natural sources of phenylethylamine (PEA). PEA is a natural mood elevator and anti-depressant. It's the same compound found in chocolate that perks-up our feel-good chemicals. However, blue-green algae has about 50 times more PEA than chocolate! It's also commonly known as the "love molecule" as it stimulates mood, feelings of overall well being, and the same euphoric feeling and feel-good chemicals that the body naturally produces during those beginning stages of falling in love. A shot of this is like being bit by the happy love bug! In addition, PEA also improves attention span, concentration, memory and the stabilization of mood swings.

HOW TO USE: Like a shot of tequila. Seriously. And be sure to have the lemon chaser ready to go as well because it tastes, well, that good. But it's SO worth it! In all honestly, it's actually not that bad, but remember to start slowly. Because it's so powerful, half an ounce should do the trick, and you can increase your dosage with time. The best way to obtain AFA is in its live, liquid state, where it's most bio-available. You'll find it frozen and it will last for five days thawed in your fridge, so defrost as you need it, or at least a couple of days' worth. If this seems a 'lil too high-maintenance for you, no need to fret, it does come in capsules as well.

> TIP: Move over chocolate — AFA will bite you with the happy love-bug. It gives you 50 times more PEA, as in the "love molecule," than chocolate.

Astragalus

Astragalus is another super-nutritious food that might not be in the display rack in your local grocery store, but totally effective when it comes to jacking-up your immune health. Astragalus is a perennial plant native to China and has been used in traditional Chinese medicine for thousands of years to strengthen the body and prevent disease. Isn't it amazing how some of the world's healthiest foods are totally under the radar in the western world? None of that. Stock up on this ancient plant your friends will be begging you for your stay-well secret!

The root is the medicinal part of astragalus and is usually harvested after four years. The root contains antiviral, antibacterial and anti-inflammatory properties, helping prevent disease and boost the immune system. It's also used to prevent colds, treat diabetes, lower blood pressure and prevent liver damage.

Similar to maca and ginseng, astragalus is an adaptogen, meaning it increases your body's response and resistance to stress. Stress is a leading cause of a suppressed immune system. You know how when you're stressed out and running off your feet, and then you *finally* get to take a vacation? Then dang!

You're sick in bed for a week, with the worst possible timing. All the stress you were under was eating away at your immune system. Stress causes inflammation and weakening of the adrenal glands, increases cortisol levels, disrupts sleep and impairs immune function. Stress also slows down and impairs the digestive process, which results in nutrients not getting absorbed and increases the toxicity of undigested food particles (which makes you feel gross and bloated, which gives you one more thing to stress about, and the vicious cycle continues). The adaptogenic properties of astragalus help reduce your body's stress response rate, strengthen the adrenals and reduce cortisol levels, all of which increase immune function. It also helps bring your body into a natural balance and state of homeostasis.

Astragalus is rich in the flavonoid quercetin, which has high antioxidant properties and can prevent against certain forms of cancer. A clinical study conducted by researchers in China suggested that supplementing astragalus with chemotherapy could inhibit the development of tumors, decrease the toxic effects of the chemo and boost the immune function and quality of life in cancer patients. In addition, the root increases phagocytosis and interferon production (trust me, these are good things), promotes T-cell maturation and increases IgA levels. The root is also rich in the minerals zinc, magnesium, silicon and iron, all of which support immune function.

HOW TO USE: So how do you get your hands on this ancient root? Astragalus is most commonly taken in supplement form and can be found in most health food stores. Traditionally in Chinese medicine, the roots of the plant were boiled and the liquid was used as a remedy, often combined with other herbs and adaptogens such as ginseng. But heads up: those with autoimmune diseases should not take astragalus, and everyone should consult with your health practitioner on a dose that's best for you.

Miso
Who knew your favorite sushi starter would be so good for you? Miso has a salty, buttery consistency and, aside from being a culinary staple in Japan for centuries, its health benefits trump its culinary applications (although it *is* super-tasty). Miso is usually fermented soy, although it can also be made from fermenting rice, wheat or barley, or a combination of the above. The soybean paste is mixed with salt and fermented using a live active (remember, this is good!) bacteria culture or a B-12 synthesizing bacteria. Miso is high in protein, B-vitamins, immune-boosting minerals and probiotics — our "friendly" bacteria.

Miso is also a rich source of zinc, which is one of the most immune-boosting minerals around. Zinc improves immune function, speeds up the healing of wounds, increases natural killer and macrophage activity and is required for the reproduction of DNA and most enzymatic processes in the body. Miso is also rich in copper and manganese, which help make up the powerhouse antioxidant superoxide dismutase (dare you to say that five times fast), which in turn is essential in fighting free-radical damage and disease. Because a bacterial form of B12 is often used in the fermenting process, miso may provide a good source of vegetarian B12 as long as it's unpasteurized. B12 is essential for a healthy immune system and disease prevention.

HOW TO USE: Whip up an easy-peasy Miso Soup (see page 163 for recipe). It takes no time at all and does wonders for your health. It's always great to have a bowl before meals to aid in digestion. It also makes an excellent salt substitute in dishes, marinades, sauces and dressings.

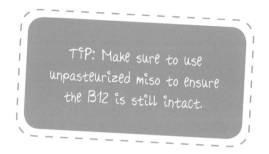

TIP: Make sure to use unpasteurized miso to ensure the B12 is still intact.

Hemp seeds

These, creamy, tiny little seeds pack a big nutritional punch. Hemp seeds are produced from the hemp plant, aka *cannabis sativa* L. But don't get too pumped, they are THC-free, and no you can't smoke them. Very different plant.

Both hemp seeds and the oil extracted from them are considered to be the perfect balance of essential fatty acids found in nature. These fats are crucial for proper brain function, heart health and digestive function, and support almost all other body systems. They are a rich source of insoluble fibre, helping to cleanse and lubricate the digestive tract. They're rich in plant-based protein, including all nine essential amino acids, and are high in key nutrients, such as B-vitamins, vitamin C, calcium, magnesium, phosphorus, potassium and iron… just to name a few.

Besides all these wicked health benefits, hemp seeds play a key role in keeping the immune system primed. About half of the hemp seed consists of a globulin known as edistin, which helps enhance the body's natural immunity. The protein from the globulin helps to give the boot to any infecting agents that may be present in the body. These little powerhouses are also rich in chlorophyll, which also detoxify the body.

Not to be outdone by our other immune boosting foods, hemp is one of the highest sources of gamma-linolenic acid (GLA), an essential fatty-acid which plays a key role in reducing disease-causing inflammation. In addition, the omega-3s and omega-6s present in hemp seeds have a slight negative charge, allowing them to carry harmful and toxic substances to the intestines, the lungs, the kidneys and the surface of skin, where they can be expelled.

HOW TO USE: The creaminess of the tiny seeds makes them an easy addition to any meal. Throw a tablespoon in your morning cereal, afternoon salad or soups. Sprinkle on top of vegetables or blend into your smoothie. You can also use hemp butter as a nut-butter substitute, hemp oil in dressings or hemp milk as a delish milk alternative. Hemp oil is a great, nutty-flavoured alternative to olive oil. It is fantastic in salad dressings or drizzled over roasted veggies. I like the blend Vega has for its Omega-3 and antioxidant profile. Hemp protein is a great addition to a smoothie as a nutrition boost. Try my delish Choco Cherry Smoothie recipe on page 135 which uses Vega Smoothie Infusion. It's a great way to get hemp protein as well as greens, Omega-3 and fibre. The little seeds also blend nicely into a chocolate macaroon crust. Check out the recipe on page 177 and I guarantee you'll be jonesing for more.

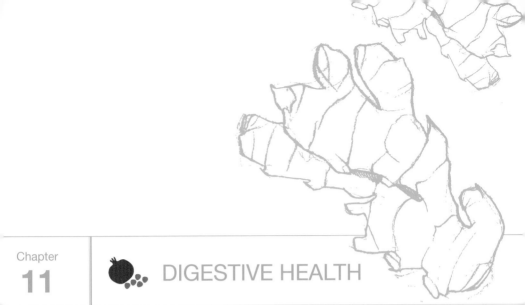

DIGESTIVE HEALTH

Damn, I'm bloated!

I love the sound of popping bubble-wrap… but not when it's coming from my stomach! Rumbles, grumbles and bloating, oh my! Not the most attractive thing, especially when accompanied by a six-inch expansion in waist circumference. Many amazing things are going on in that tummy of yours. It's where the magic happens. Food gets broken down and nutrients get absorbed. Your health, your thoughts, your weight, everything we talk about in this book is connected to not just what you eat, but how you assimilate your food and nutrients. Remember, 80 per cent of your immune system resides in your gut. Listen to what it's telling you and it will thank you by keeping you feeling your best!

Poor digestion

Sometimes we wake up with a nice flat tummy but by the end of the day we may look six months pregnant! While overactive and underactive stomach can both cause tummy troubles, sometimes the causes are not quite as straightforward. Poor food combining, inadequate digestive enzymes, low stomach acid (HCl), not enough 'good' bacteria or food sensitivities are typically the problem.

WHAT TO DO?

Probiotics are live microorganisms classified as good bacteria that help fight off all the bad bacteria. They improve digestion and help your body assimilate the precious vitamins and nutrients within your food keeping you healthy. There is 20 times more bacteria in your body than the actual billions of cells that make up your body – make sure you're sporting the 'good' kind! To help the good guys win, try noshing on coconut kefir, miso soup, raw sauerkraut, kombucha and yogurt.

Digestive enzymes also helps to breakdown food and assimilate nutrients. Look for digestive enzymes that contain HCl which will help to breakdown food including fibre and plant roughage. This will also aid in digestion of protein as the enzyme pepsin is only activated in the presence of HCl. Pop your digestive enzymes about 12-15 minutes before a meal to help the digestive process.

Elimination diets can help to rule out food sensitivities. Try cutting out common allergen foods, such as dairy, soy, wheat, gluten, eggs and peanuts for a minimum of two weeks and then one-by-one, start adding each of the foods back in, taking note of how you feel. And if symptoms re-occur, you've found your culprit!

Let's take a look at the two most common digestive issues — an underactive stomach and an overactive stomach.

Underactive stomach

An underactive stomach is one of the most common digestive complaints. Many people confuse it with an overactive stomach and take antacids as a result — which makes the condition even worse! An underactive stomach is one that does not produce enough hydrochloric acid (HCl). Hydrochloric acid is released in the stomach to break down food, including fibre and plant roughage. In addition, the enzyme pepsin, which is used to digest protein, is only activated in the presence of HCl.

HCl also works to protect the body from harmful microorganisms such as bad bacteria, parasites and viruses. It encourages the production of enzymes and the absorption of vitamins and minerals. In particular, calcium, iron and zinc require adequate levels of HCl in the stomach in order to be metabolized and absorbed.

HCl naturally declines with age. However, the following factors also aggravate the condition:
- Diet high in red meat
- Dairy products
- Refined and processed foods
- Drinking too much fluids with meals
- Poor food combining
- Not chewing your food
- Emotional stress
- Eating too quickly

The symptoms of HCl-deficiency can include:
- Excessive gas, belching or burping after meals
- Constipation
- Stomach bloated after eating
- Halitosis

- Feeling too full after a heavy-meat meal
- Heavy, tired feeling after eating
- Nausea after taking supplements
- Dry skin, acne
- Undigested food in stool
- Poor absorption of nutrients/malnourishment

How to combat an underactive stomach

1 *Digestive Enzymes.* Take four or five digestive enzymes immediately before a meal. This helps break down food and assimilate nutrients. Try to purchase digestive enzymes that contain HCl.

2 *Slow down.* Don't eat when rushed, anxious or stressed. This will only aggravate the condition.

3 *Chew your food!* The digestion of carbohydrates begins in your mouth! Amylase, which breaks down carbs, is secreted through your saliva gland. So the longer you munch away on your food, not only will you be breaking down the particles into smaller pieces, making it easier for your body to digest, but you will kick-start the digestive process right in your chomper! See those teeth? They aren't there just to look pretty… use those pearly whites and chew, chew, chew till your food is liquid!

4 *Don't drink with meals.* Drinking with meals flushes away those precious digestive enzymes. Drink at least 30 minutes before your meal or two hours after your meal for optimal digestion.

5 *Apple cider vinegar.* Acidic foods such as apple cider vinegar can help stimulate HCl. Try taking one tablespoon before a meal or add to salads. If you take apple cider vinegar with your meals and your symptoms dissipate, it's because you have low stomach acid. If they worsen, you have high stomach acid (see the next section on an overactive stomach).

6 *Try an elimination and rotation diet.* Food sensitivities can cause inflammation of your intestinal tract, impeding the digestive process and preventing the assimilation of nutrients — and causing serious boating! Try cutting out major allergens (such as wheat, gluten, dairy and soy) for minimum of two weeks and slowly add these foods back in, one by one, taking note of how you feel. I guarantee during that two-week window you'll feel fab and your tummy will feel tight!

7 *Practice food combining.* Different foods digest at different rates. Melon may take only 30 minutes to digest, whereas a steak can take four hours! Follow the simple principles below and you should notice your symptoms improve.

Food combining

Proper assimilation of food requires the use of digestive enzymes. Different types of food require different digestive enzymes. The human body is not designed to digest more than one type of food in the stomach at the same time, nor can it manufacture all the necessary enzymes simultaneously. Some foods, such as melons, digest in less than 30 minutes, whereas nuts can take up to four hours. Eating these types of food together cause stress on your digestive system.

The results of poor food combining include:
- Bloating
- Weight gain
- Indigestion
- Poor assimilation of nutrients
- Lack of energy
- Toxic waste build-up

Combinations to *avoid*:
- Starch + protein — creates various gases in your system, including sulfur
- Starch + fruit — creates fermentation and alcohol
- Protein + fruit — produces a variety of toxic by-products

Combinations to *follow*:
- Leafy greens and vegetables + proteins
- Leafy greens and vegetables + fats
- Leafy greens and vegetables + starches
- Fruit and sweet foods should be eaten alone
- Avocados combine well with almost everything (protein, fruit, vegetables, leafy greens) but do not combine well with starch

Protein 4 hours to digest	Starch 3 hours to digest	Vegetables 2.5 hours to digest	Fruit 2 hours to digest
Nuts Seeds Fish/meat Milks (nut, hemp)	Grains Beans & legumes Winter squash Potatoes, sweet potatoes and yams	Sprouts Leafy greens Cucumber Peppers Summer squash Broccoli Cabbage Cauliflower Corn Root vegetables (carrots, beets, parsnips)	All fruit, including tomatoes *Melons take 15-30 minutes to digest and should not be combined with any other fruit*

Overactive stomach

An overactive stomach occurs when your body produces too much HCL.
Typically, this may be associated with an ulcer or lesion in the intestinal lining.

Here's how to tell if your tummy is overacting:
- Stomach pain one hour after eating or at night
- Burning sensation in stomach
- Pain aggravated by worry/tension
- Hiatal hernia, gastritis, gastric ulcer
- Nausea, vomiting
- Sensation of acidity in abdominal area
- Lower back pain
- Blood in stool

The causes of an overactive stomach can include a diet rich in spicy foods, long-term use of aspirin, or a diet rich in caffeine, alcohol, tobacco, sugars and nitrates. One of the best foods to treat an overactive stomach? Aloe vera. See page 95 for more on this tummy-calming food!

FOODS TO AID IN DIGESTIVE HEALTH

Whether your stomach is overactive or underactive, here are a few key foods that will help your tummy return to a happy, healthy state of being.

Ginger
You might think of ginger as a common spice in Indian or Asian cooking, but don't be fooled by its boring beige colour — ginger is anything but bland! This powerful herb, spice, nutritional supplement and medicinal healer has been used all over the world since ancient times for much more than just spicing up dishes (and cookies!).

Ginger's effects as a digestive miracle worker are by far its most impressive qualities. For thousands of years, Chinese doctors have used ginger to manage nausea, vomiting, diarrhea and stomach upset. Your mom was onto something when she made you drink flat ginger ale for an upset tummy. Ginger helps relieve indigestion, gas pains, diarrhea and stomach cramping by increasing the production of digestive fluids and saliva. The relief ginger provides from nausea caused by morning sickness or motion sickness is by far its most highly-acclaimed action in the body. Studies have shown its anti-nausea properties are significantly more effective than Dramamine in curbing motion sickness. A double-blind randomized trial done at Thammasat University in Thailand studied the effects of either one gram of ginger in capsule form taken daily or 100 milligrams of Dimenhydrinate (Dramamine) on 170 women experiencing nausea and vomiting during pregnancy. The results showed that ginger is equally effective in the treatment of nausea and vomiting during pregnancy, and has fewer side effects.

Ginger has many other health properties as well. It is a known diaphoretic, meaning it causes you to sweat, and is perfect to help break a fever and detoxify the body when excess toxins are present. It is a natural anti-inflammatory, and is often used as a therapeutic and natural remedy for sufferers of arthritis and rheumatism. It has properties that stimulate circulation of the blood, remove toxins from the body, cleanse the kidneys and strengthen bowel function. Bonus: ginger is believed to have aphrodisiac powers and is even mentioned in the Kama Sutra. Its ability to protect against symptoms of the common cold and flu also make it a fantastic preventative measure when your immune system needs a boost. On top of all that, ginger lowers cholesterol and acts as an antioxidant and antihistamine, improving symptoms of allergies. Ginger root is also useful for respiratory problems, helping to rid the lungs of phlegm.

HOW TO USE: In his book *Perfect Digestion*, author Deepak Chopra recommends a drink of ginger and lemon to kindle the digestive fire while helping to tone the digestive tract. Consuming ginger in the form of tea, either fresh or dried, is an easy and delicious way to get your digestive juice flowing. Ginger in cooking isn't necessarily enough to kindle that digestive flame, so if you need some substantial digestive support, try a ginger capsule daily. This all-around health-booster will work wonders for your digestion and assimilation (and maybe even your libido!).

Licorice
Licorice is best known for giving that distinct, sweet and much-loved taste to its popular candy counterpart, but most people remain highly unaware of what a powerful herb licorice root is in supporting whole body health. This naturally sweet and delicious herb has been used for medicinal healing in China since ancient times, and is considered to be among the most important healing herbs in the practice of traditional Chinese medicine. It got its name from the Greek word for "sweet root," and has been used for thousands of years as a flavouring and intense sweetener.

Licorice's demulcent action is the reason it is praised as a wonder herb to help calm and support digestive health. It does this by coating the mucus membrane with a soothing film that helps to alleviate pain and inflammation, while also protecting the integrity of the stomach and intestinal walls and supporting smooth digestive tract function. A form of licorice, deglycyrrhizinated licorice (DGL), is a natural supplement often used to treat ulcers (both gastric and duodenal) with great success. Licorice is believed to promote the healing of the digestive tissues in cases of ulceration by stimulating the protective lining of the stomach. An endoscopic study of 32 cases of duodenal ulceration treated with DGL tablets daily showed that significant healing of the ulceration had occurred, and in the majority of cases, the mucosa appeared normal.

All stuffed up? Licorice can help clear those clogged airways! Licorice contains a compound called glycyrrhizin, which has anti-inflammatory properties. Licorice root has an expectorant effect in the body, helping keep your lungs clear and treating respiratory troubles. These expectorant properties help loosen phlegm in the body and can ease coughs, congestion and colds. The antibacterial action of the glycyrrhetinic acid in licorice can halt the growth of many bacteria and further support the respiratory tract in fighting infection, so that slight cough doesn't turn into something more nasty. Acting as an antiviral, licorice also helps fight off viruses such as the flu and hepatitis B.

In recent years, herbalists have also been using licorice to combat adrenal weakness, which can be caused by a combination of stress and poor diet. The herb contains a natural hormone that stimulates increased production of cortisone and aldosterone, helping the body better cope with excess stress and exhaustion while boosting energy levels at the same time. Licorice root is also considered an herbal alterative, a cleansing stimulant that is effective in removing toxins and wastes from the body. It promotes cleansing of the colon and is also used to purify the liver, which is the body's center for detoxification.

HOW TO USE: Thinking of heading down to the corner store for some licorice laces? Think again! There are way more effective ways you can add licorice to your diet without the empty calories. Licorice can be taken regularly for maintenance of healthy digestion in tea, or can be taken in the form of DGL capsules for therapeutic purposes. If you think licorice could work to help you balance your digestive processes, bear in mind that contraindications include women who are pregnant or nursing, and those with high blood pressure. Otherwise, let this nutritious and tasty herb do its thing!

Apple cider vinegar

Vinegar is a pretty typical culinary condiment. Apple cider vinegar, however, is produced slightly differently than other vinegars and has many more health benefits than your run-of-the-mill supermarket vinegar. Apple cider vinegar is made by crushing apples to produce a liquid. Sugar and yeast are added to this liquid, which is then matured in wooden barrels. These barrels help to boost fermentation much more than in other distilled grocery store vinegars, and this process turns the sugars into alcohol, which is then converted (by an acetic acid-forming bacteria) into vinegar.

When the vinegar is "mature," there is a dark and cloudy bacteria present called the "mother" of vinegar. It is a term used to refer to the mass of scum that forms on top of cider when alcohol turns into vinegar, which is actually bacteria and yeast cells that have died. I know — totally gross. Although this doesn't sounds very appetizing, natural vinegars that contain the mother have extremely high levels of enzymes and minerals that other vinegars do not. It is a natural bacteria-fighting substance that contains many vital nutrients and minerals to support a healthy body. It is for this reason that apple cider vinegar is believed to have so many health benefits. So… just promise you won't think about how it's made and reap the benefits, 'kay?

You'd be surprised at some of the things apple cider vinegar is used for! Some of its common uses are for weight loss, acne, yeast infections, constipation and diarrhea. Heading out on the town? It is also used to combat bad breath, body odour and cellulite. It's even suggested for diabetics to help regulate blood sugar levels.

One of the most commonly-acknowledged uses for this powerful vinegar is in balancing acid levels in the stomach to facilitate proper digestion. As we age, it is common for our bodies to produce less stomach acid. This decrease in hydrochloric acid can lead to digestive problems, especially sensations of heartburn and stomach upset. Although heartburn is commonly accepted in the medical world as a problem of excess acid in the stomach, the reality is that acid reflux can also be a product of diminished stomach acid.

HOW TO USE: By taking a little apple cider vinegar in water before every meal, you can enhance the stomach acid production and increase digestive enzyme function. It can also improve digestion, assimilation and nutrient uptake, while having an overall alkalinizing effect on the body. Taking two to three tablespoons in water before meals can increase digestive function and help re-balance the gut ecology. And like many of these healthy-but-not-necessarily-tasty remedies, you can always take it as a shooter if that helps it go down!

Peppermint

This leaf works magic in a mojito, or in mint chocolate chunk ice cream… or in a creative combo of the two, if that's how roll! But you might want to save a few leaves to work their magic on your tummy, post nosh. Peppermint tea is recognized around the world for its wide range of medicinal benefits in the body, but it is most loved and appreciated for the wonderful effect it has on our digestive system.

Apart from its distinct and delicious taste, peppermint's herbal properties include anti-spasmotic, antiseptic, antiemetic (relieving vomiting) and acting as a nervine tonic to relax the central nervous system. Peppermint is also an effective carminative, which soothes the stomach and intestinal wall, relaxing and calming our digestive tract and relieving cramping.

The active ingredient in peppermint leaf is menthol, a volatile oil with very powerful therapeutic properties. Menthol acts as a mild analgesic, which relieves nausea, vomiting, travel sickness and morning sickness. Bloated? It's relaxing effects on the muscles surrounding the digestive system help relieve gas (in a way that won't clear the room). It also promotes digestive function by stimulating the release of bile and the flow of digestive juices in the stomach and intestines. In fact, peppermint oil can even play a role in treating more severe digestive disorders, such as ulcerative colitis, Crohn's disease and irritable bowel syndrome.

And don't think peppermint tea is just for digestion! It's good for what ails you if you want to strengthen your immune system, jack-up on vitamin C, kibosh a pounding headache, or just chill after a long day.

HOW TO USE: Make yourself a soothing peppermint tea or blend some peppermint with chocolate hemp milk for a nutri'licious minty smoothie. Or go straight to the source and chew on some leaves to freshen breath and aid in digestion.

> TIP: If you are feeling constipated, try combining peppermint tea with a magnesium supplement to get things moving again!

Kombucha

Move over Veuve. There's a new bubbly in town. 'Kay, maybe not so new — this vintage living health drink has been used for thousands of years balance and harmonize the body. Kombucha is a fermented tea referred to as the Tea of Immortality and the Elixir of Life. But just how does kombucha support total health and vitality?

The kombucha culture is a mushroom, often called the "mother" or SCOBY, which stands for "symbiotic culture of bacteria and yeasts." The culture is placed in black or green tea and turns the sweet tea into a delicious and naturally bubbly beverage packed with vitamins, minerals, enzymes and health-promoting organic acids. As the kombucha culture digests the sugar, it produces a range of organic acids including glucuronic acid and lactic acid. It also produces B-vitamins and vitamin C, as well as amino acids and enzymes. On top of all of these health-supporting nutrients, the SCOBY itself is filled with a plethora of probiotic microorganisms to support all body systems.

The probiotics present in the SCOBY are one of the main reasons kombucha is such a fantastic digestive tonic. Probiotics are good bacteria that keep our digestive system balanced. As a probiotic, kombucha aids the stomach in the breakdown and digestion of food, preventing acid reflux and relieving constipation. The good bacteria and yeast present in the drink reduce bad bacteria and parasites in the gut, which is why kombucha can be effective in the treatment of candida, an increasingly common overgrowth of yeast in the body.

The synergism of the stomach acid and the fermented kombucha is thought to cause the formation of an alkaline substance in the digestive tract, which aids in the proper functioning of all body organs, particularly the spleen, intestines, gall bladder and pancreas. Impressive, but that's not all. This power drink is often used for its energy-boosting properties, can improve metabolism and support healthy weight loss, and has detox properties. Cheers to that!

Other health properties include antibiotic, antifungal and antiviral characteristics, which allow our bodies to fight off bacteria, viruses, and all other foreign invaders they come up against. Kombucha is thought to improve hypertension, allergies, chronic fatigue and especially arthritis. There are even those who believe it has a part to play in the treatment of HIV and cancer.

HOW TO USE: You can find kombucha bottled up and ready to drink in the fridge of most health food stores. Pour some in a champagne flute and enjoy with your meal or on its own. You can make a kombucha float using kombucha and my Banana Pear Ice Kreme recipe on page 183 or make fun cocktails. And hey, if you want to throw a little vodka in there, I won't tell. It also makes a great hangover remedy, FYI. If you're feeling adventurous, you can even make kombucha yourself at home in approximately two weeks of fermenting, so get brewing! Its funky fermented taste may take a little getting used to, but both the physical and mental effects are highly-addictive. Drink responsibly.

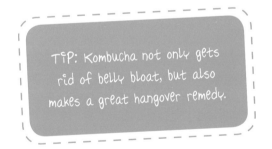

TIP: Kombucha not only gets rid of belly bloat, but also makes a great hangover remedy.

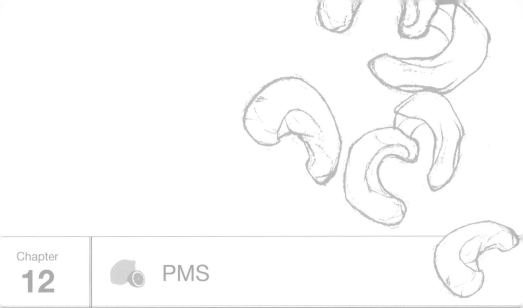

Chapter		
12		PMS

Please Make it Stop — PMS, or premenstrual syndrome that is! This is the period (pun intended) where your cool, fun-loving, normal self turns into psycho-chick. For real. But it's totally excusable. You're boobs hurt just running down the stairs, all your clothes immediately become tight, you never know when that zit is about to pop up on your face, and you can barely get out of bed in the morning, coupled with the fact that you couldn't even fall asleep. You may feel tense, irritated, irrational, bloated, crampy, achy, cranky, sad, moody and hungry for all the wrong foods. Yep — pretty much hell. What's worse is that an estimated three out of four women actually report having these feelings. It's no wonder men don't understand us.

PMS FACTS: CHECK YOURSELF BEFORE YOU WRECK YOURSELF

The good news? You're not losing your mind when you burst into tears for no apparent reason. Mood swings, fatigue and depression are common feelings you might experience during PMS. Another number to note? 200. That's the number of different symptoms that have been associated with PMS, and since there isn't enough room to list them all here, the three most commonly reported are feelings of unhappiness, cramps and mood swings that bring on wicked food cravings. If it's greasy, sugary, salty, fatty and starchy, it may end up on your plate because the body is trying to compensate and correct the hormonal gong show that is your body. And it totally takes over all control. You've lost all sense of reason and it feels as though there is nothing you can do. But that's not necessarily true. Current thinking suggests that estrogen excess, progesterone deficiencies, vitamin B6 deficiencies, low levels of serotonin, and low calcium could explain PMS. And what you eat a couple of weeks before your period could significantly reduce PMS, or better yet, PCS (psycho-chick syndrome).

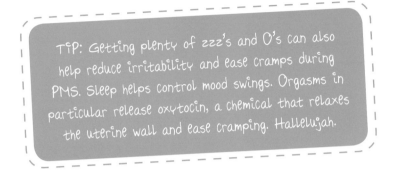

TIP: Getting plenty of zzz's and O's can also help reduce irritability and ease cramps during PMS. Sleep helps control mood swings. Orgasms in particular release oxytocin, a chemical that relaxes the uterine wall and ease cramping. Hallelujah.

PMS-FIGHTING NUTRIENTS

Calcium, magnesium and vitamin D

The similarity in symptoms between low calcium levels and PMS is strong. Calcium absorption fluctuates across the menstrual cycle, since estrogen levels also change. It has been determined that estrogen regulates calcium metabolism. In one study from the Columbia University College of Physicians and Surgeons, women who received 1,200 milligrams of calcium carbonate each day for three menstrual cycles had a 50 per cent reduction in PMS symptoms. The equation is easy. Up the intake of calcium, and reduce the cramping and pains associated with PMS. Magnesium is one of the top mineral deficiencies at any time of the month, and it's especially important to supplement during PMS because it helps relax nerves and alleviate muscle cramping and headaches. The hype around consuming vitamin D during PMS is also significant. Dubbed the sunshine vitamin, vitamin D helps the body absorb calcium. Since calcium helps ease cramping, pairing your calcium with vitamin D can maximize the cramp-curbing benefits. Later, cramps.

TIP: Since PMS is closely linked to estrogen dominance, the same principals apply. See chapter 6 for more info.

Omega 3 fatty acids and GLA

Essential fatty acids (EFAs) are an essential BFF when it comes to PMS. Why? Well, EFAs play important roles in your body's overall health. They are part of every cell and establish and control the cellular metabolism. Omega-3 EFAs are great for their anti-inflammatory properties, and they also provide energy, maintain body temperature, insulate our nerves and cushion and protect body tissues. Gamma linolenic acid (GLA) also provides amazing anti-inflammatory properties, and in particular, forms other substances such as prostaglandins. Prostaglandins are hormone-like substances, vital chemicals that regulate heartbeat and blood pressure. They also play a role in breaking up cholesterol deposits in the blood. Most importantly, they help alleviate cramping and backaches during PMS because of the anti-inflammatory properties.

Vitamin B6

B-vitamins in general are great for PMS, but B6 in particular is essential in the production of those feel-good neurotransmitters. It helps in the conversion of tryptophan to serotonin, and who doesn't love the high you get off of that? Unfortunately, this vitamin is also the first to be depleted during times of tension, so a lack of B6 could seriously lead to more feelings of depression. We know that PMS makes us feel like crap, so you can see why it's so important to keep taking that B6 during the day and keep elevating those serotonin levels. Take 100 milligrams of vitamin B6 a day, combined with other B vitamins, and go to your happy place!

> TIP: What you eat up to two weeks before your period can make a HUGE difference when it comes to PMS. Try to incorporate more PMS-busting foods and eliminate PMS-promoting foods, such as dairy, refined carbs, sugars and alcohols.

Indole-3-carbinol

Indole-3-carbinol or I3C might not be easy to pronounce, but it's a phytochemical that you want to remember to incorporate in your diet during PMS. It's a strong antioxidant, but most importantly it helps shift estrogen metabolism to less estrogenic metabolites. Especially during PMS, it helps maintain hormonal balance and can relive muscle soreness.

Fibre

Fibre is the new black. It does everything from lowering cholesterol to normalizing blood sugar and in turn reducing food cravings. It also removes excess estrogen from the body, which is crucial for helping ease PMS symptoms. If estrogen is not eliminated properly, it can be reactivated while in the liver and actually re-enter the blood stream, causing hormonal chaos to ensue. Fibre also helps the body fully utilize progesterone, which if in excess, can cause food cravings to rocket. To balance the blood sugar levels fluctuating during PMS, the body releases adrenaline, but if it's not utilized progesterone is not used efficiently. Fibre helps to balance this by eliminating progesterone as waste. It's recommended that adults consume 20 to 35 grams of dietary fibre per day.

Kale

Killer cramps? Curb them with kale. Kale is a dense green leafy vegetable that comes from the cabbage family. Whether it's green or purple, curly or plain-leaved, kale is one of the perfect foods to help during PMS because it contains calcium, magnesium, I3C and calcium d-glucarate.

Calcium is the simplest and least expensive intervention for PMS. A clinical study involving 497 women at St. Luke's-Roosevelt Hospital in New York found taking 1,200 milligrams of calcium carbonate daily led to a lessening of fluid retention, food cravings and pain after three months. Aim for 1,200 milligrams of calcium per day to help with cramps. The I3C helps to weaken estrogen levels while the calcium d-glucarate, coupled with the fibre, helps eliminate excess estrogen from your body, making you less estrogenic, significantly reducing the severity of PMS. No more yo-yo hormones for you. In addition, kale is a natural diuretic, helping to eliminate excess water weight!

HOW TO USE: Often relegated as a salad bar garnish, this hearty green has oh-so-much-more to offer. Try adding it to a salad filled with other leafy greens. Kale has a crunchier bite and offers a great balance of textures. Or try lightly steaming kale and toss with olive oil, black pepper and sea salt for a side dish that adds colour and nutrition. Slice it up with a bunch of other veggies for a delish stir fry. In season in early winter, kale makes a hearty addition to soups or stews. But my all-time fave — and soon to be yours — are kale chips. All you have to do is slice kale leaves into bite size pieces, removing the stems. Toss in some olive oil, lemon juice and paprika and then dehydrates or bake on low. The result: a salty, crunchy substitute to potato chips, loaded with nutrition and free of guilt!

Halibut

Halibut is your anti-cramping BFF. Halibut is rich in omega-3 fatty acids, which slow down the release of prostaglandins. Prostaglandins regulate pain and inflammation in the body. By managing prostaglandin release with Omega-3s, you can reduce pain in the joints, lower back, abdomen and headaches. For these reasons, Omega-3s may also reduce breast tenderness, mood changes and weight gain. Halibut is also a rich source of magnesium, which helps relax nerves and tense muscles and relieves cramping.

HOW TO USE: Forget the standard fare of fish and chips, halibut's mild flavour lends itself to grilling and baking perfectly, without the added saturated fat. Be sure to buy fresh, wild halibut for optimum nutrition profile. Halibut is great and most nutritious when baked, steamed or grilled; your fish is cooked through when opaque. Remember not to overcook or you're looking at a dry, flavorless mess. Halibut pairs well with a variety of herbs; dill, rosemary and parsley are all great complements. Try experimenting with this Omega-3 star by adding to a sprouted grain wrap with veggies or toss into your favourite soup or pasta.

Maca

Maca is definitely a PMS-busting superfood. It's nutrient-dense, hormone-balancing, stress-busting properties will make that time of the month a stroll in the park for you – and everyone around you! Maca is a rich source of I-3-C which helps change excess bad estrogen into a weaker, beneficial form. And since hormonal imbalances and estrogen dominance typically lead to weight-gain, cramping, mood-swings and bitchiness, maca is a must. Plus it's rich fibre content helps to pull the excess estrogen, preventing it from re-circulating. Maca is also rich in calcium and magnesium to help relieve killer cramps.

HOW TO USE: Discover the many ways to use maca on page 42.

Sacha inchi seeds

Omega-3 is key when to reducing inflammation, stomach cramping and regulating mood. Sacha inchi seeds (SaviSeed) are among the richest source, helping you feel fab. Plus at five grams of fibre per ounce, it will help balance blood sugar levels, ward off wicked cravings and keep energy levels stable.

HOW TO USE: Learn how to incorporate sacha inchi seeds into your diet on page 52.

Quinoa

Pronounced "keen-wa," this is one of my favourite carbs. A nutritional powerhouse, quinoa is renowned for its protein content (at 12 to 18 percent protein, quinoa contains all nine essential amino acids). Classified as a pseudograin, quinoa is a seed that cooks like rice. Substitute it for other grains or toss it in a salad for an extra protein punch that's easier to digest than animal protein, with more vitamins and minerals and far lower fat content.

Quinoa is also gluten-free, full of fibre and contains copious amounts of nutrients, including B vitamins. B vitamins and fibre are crucial for helping balance hormones. B vitamins are essential in the production of serotonin, which helps reduce irritability, depression, and PCS (phycho-chick syndrome). Fibre reduces cravings to binge because it bulks up in the stomach so you feel fuller longer. This also helps eliminate excess estrogen, balancing hormones and reducing water retention. When estrogen starts to fluctuate, it affects aldosterone, a hormone that affects the way your kidneys hold on to water. This is why you retain more water during PMS. So by noshing on quinoa, your excess water weight starts to normalize and there will be zero need to bust out your "fat clothes."

HOW TO USE: I love quinoa not only because it's so nutri'licious, but because it's also super low-maintenance! It only takes 15 minutes to cook and last in your fridge cooked for up to five days, making it a quick and easy meal, no matter what your time constraints are. Use it as a base of a pasta dish, as a rice substitute, blended into soups or smoothies, used in a salad, as a breakfast cereal, or in cookies. Yep, that's right. Check out my PMS-busting are my Quinoa Cookies on page 181.

Raw cashews
Raw cashews are the perfect PMS-busting snack food. They're rammed with essential vitamins, minerals and nutrients that support regulating mood, food cravings and relaxing muscles. Some of the most important PMS-busting nutrients include magnesium, vitamin B, vitamin E and and fibre. Cashews are loaded in magnesium, a powerful nutrient to support nervous system function. High levels of magnesium support a relaxed mind and body, which helps alleviate cramping. Magnesium also activates many enzymes required for energy production in the body, which is key when you are fatigued. As B-vitamins and magnesium are both involved in the production of serotonin, they can further help regulate mood and relieve bitchiness.

Cashews also make a great snack because they can help keep blood-sugar levels in check, reducing killer cravings and binges. According to studies conducted through the University of Montreal and Université de Yaoundé cashew seed extract significantly stimulated blood sugar absorption by muscle cells. This not only helps to keep energy levels, mood, and cravings in check, but can help prevent insulin resistance, type 2 diabetes, and most importantly, prevent your mid-section from bulging over your jeans! Buh-bye PCS and muffin tops, hello hot chick!

HOW TO USE: To knock out PMS, reach for raw, unroasted, unsalted cashews. (And no, that doesn't take all the fun out it!) These little nuts are a rich addition to salads, cereal, and baked goods but keep in mind that these babies are high in fat and calories so moderation is the way to go. Also, they are not the highest quality of nut. Make sure you get them from a reputable source as they can have mold content; especially troublesome if you suffer from candida. These days you can also find cashew butter on store shelves, a great alternative to traditional peanut butter. I love using them in my guilt-free desserts. Try my Choco Mocha Mousse Cup or Lemon Berry Tart recipes (on page 179 and 185 respectively) to see what I mean. Delici-o-so!

TiP: Top PMS-busting foods — Cruciferous veggies, Maca, Chia seeds, Sacha inchi seeds, Hemp seeds, Bananas, Cucumber, Almonds, Raw chocolate, Dark leafy greens, Apples, Quinoa, Oats.

section 5

RECIPES

Create drinks, appies, soups, salads, entrees and desserts to put it everything you've learned into practice!.

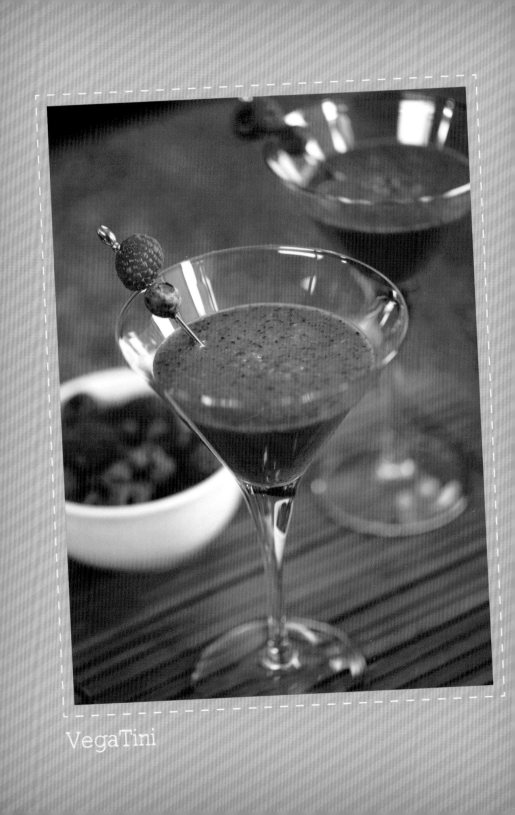

VegaTini

VegaTini

This is the best hangover cocktail remedy EVER!!! It lets you party like a rock star and still feel fab. It helps to re-hydrate, replenish precious vitamins and minerals, detox your liver and reduce nausea that usually follows a night of indulgence.

- 2 ½ cups coconut water
- 1 scoop Vega Whole Food Health Optimizer – berry
- 2" cube fresh ginger
- 1 tbsp camu camu powder
- 1 cup frozen blueberries
- 2" piece frozen banana
- Squeeze of ½ lemon

Add all ingredients to blender and combine thoroughly.

WHY THIS WORKS?
Coconut water rich in electrolytes to re-hydrate and replenish precious minerals that have been lost and antioxidants to prevent all the free-radical damaged caused by alcohol. The Vega Whole Food Health Optimizer will help your liver detox the alcohol, keep blood sugar in check and prevent a killer hangover. The ginger gets rid of room-spins and nausea and also helps to cleanse and reduce liver inflammation. The camu camu and blueberries are rich in vitamin C, which helps to break down and metabolize blood alcohol. And the squeeze of lemon… so your liver doesn't totally hate your guts for all the abuse!

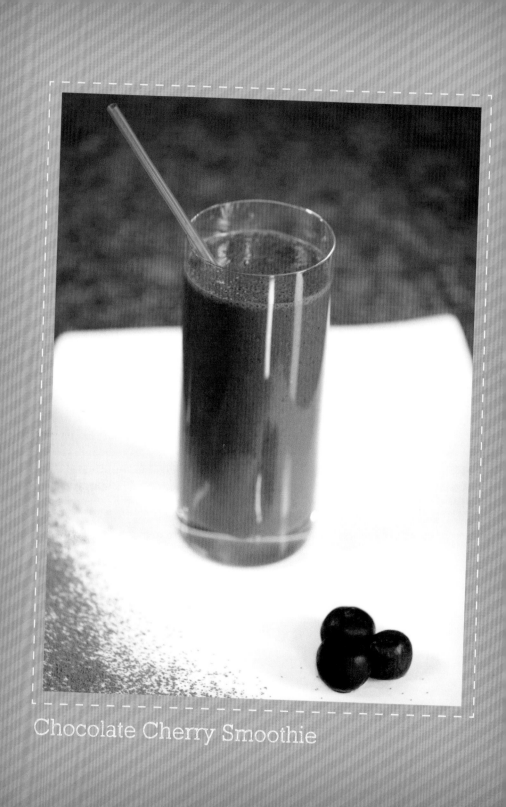

Chocolate Cherry Smoothie

Chocolate Cherry Smoothie

After a hard day, this 'calming' combination of chocolate and cherry is so delish it will melt all your worries away, taking you into a state of pure bliss!

- 2 cups hemp milk
- 1 cup frozen tart cherries (or ½ cup tart cherry juice and ½ cup cherries)
- 3 tbsp raw cacao powder
- 1 tbsp cacao nibs
- 1 pinch ground cinnamon
- 1 scoop Vega Smoothie Infusion
- Seeds from pod of one vanilla bean or ¼ tsp pure vanilla extract
- ½ tsp yacon syrup

Add all ingredients to blender and combine thoroughly.

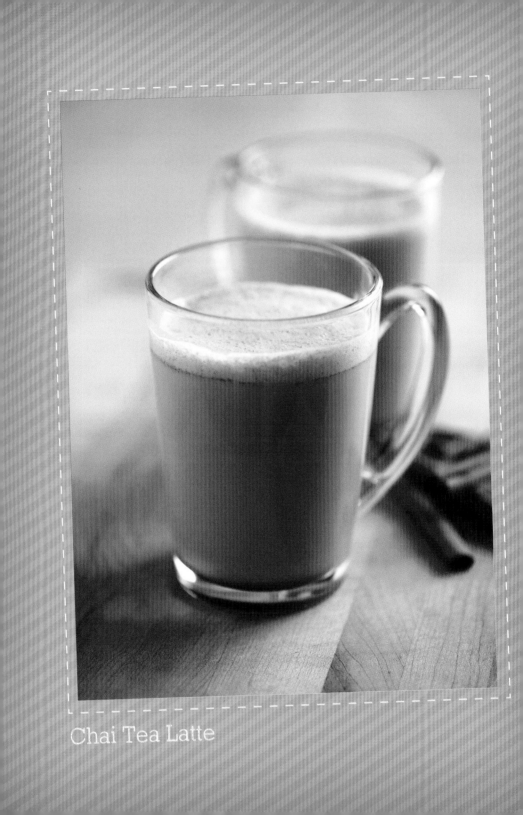

Chai Tea Latte

Chai Tea Latte

A big cup of comfort… Good after a meal or in-between meals to satisfy both a sugar or coffee craving. It's like a big hug from the inside out!

- 1 Rooibos chai tea bag
- 1 tbsp almond butter
- 1 cup boiling water
- ¼ tsp ground cinnamon
- ¼ tsp vanilla extract
- Pinch ground cardamom (optional)
- Pinch ground nutmeg (optional)

Steep tea in boiling water for about 5 minutes and remove bag. Add tea to blender with almond butter, cinnamon and vanilla. Blend into a creamy latte. Garnish latte with a pinch of cardamom and /or nutmeg. Serves one.

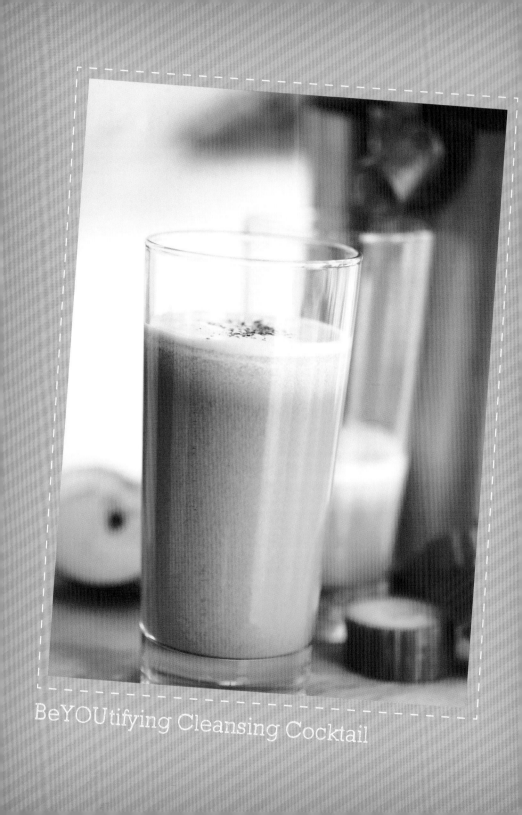

BeYOUtifying Cleansing Cocktail

BeYOUtifying Cleansing Cocktail

Get amazingly glowing skin from the inside-out with this simple and delicious cocktail! And it might just help you get rid of belly-bloat and drop a few pounds too!

- 3 large stalks celery
- 1 cucumber
- 2 apples
- 2 ½" cube fresh ginger
- Juice from ½ lemon
- Pinch cayenne pepper

Juice celery, cucumber, apples and ginger. Stir in lemon juice. Pour into glass and add pinch of cayenne. Stir, enjoy and feel your skin glow!

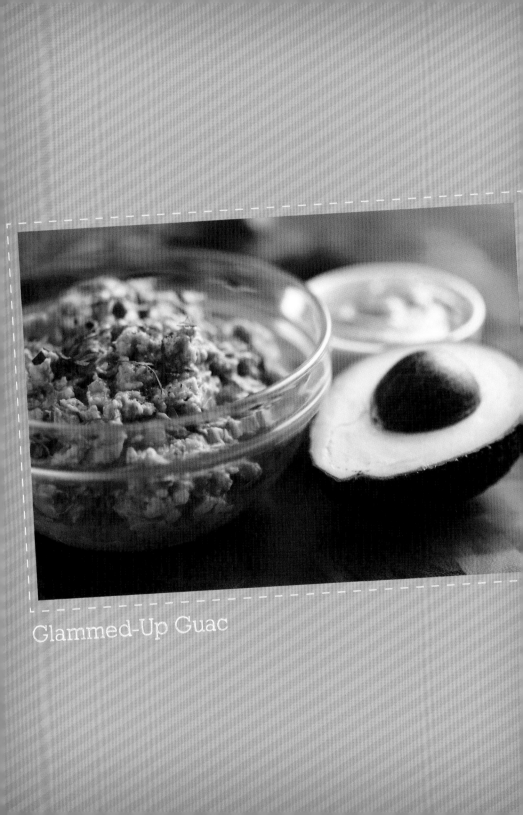

Glammed-Up Guac

Glammed-Up Guac

Get glam and glowing with this beautifying appetizer. Super rich in vitamin E and healthy fats, avocados are great for moisturizing your skin from the inside out.

GUACAMOLE:
- 3 ripe avocados
- 1 tbsp chipotle peppers, finely diced
- ½ Spanish onion, finely diced
- 1 clove garlic, finely diced
- ⅓ cup fresh cilantro leaves, chopped
- Juice of ½ lemon
- Juice of 1 lime
- 1 tsp ground cumin
- ½ tsp ground coriander
- ¼ tsp chilli powder
- Cayenne pepper (optional)
- ¼ tsp sea salt

Remove flesh of avocado and add to a bowl. Mash coarsely with a fork. Mix in all remaining ingredients. Garnish with cayenne pepper and sea salt to taste.

CHIPOTLE KREME:
- ¾ cup raw cashews
- 1 tbsp pureed chipotle peppers
- 1 small clove garlic, minced
- ½ cup water

Add all ingredients high powder blender and blend into a smooth puree.

SERVING SUGGESTION:
- 4 heads Belgian endive

Serve Guacamole on Belgian endive leaves with a drizzle of Chipotle Kreme.

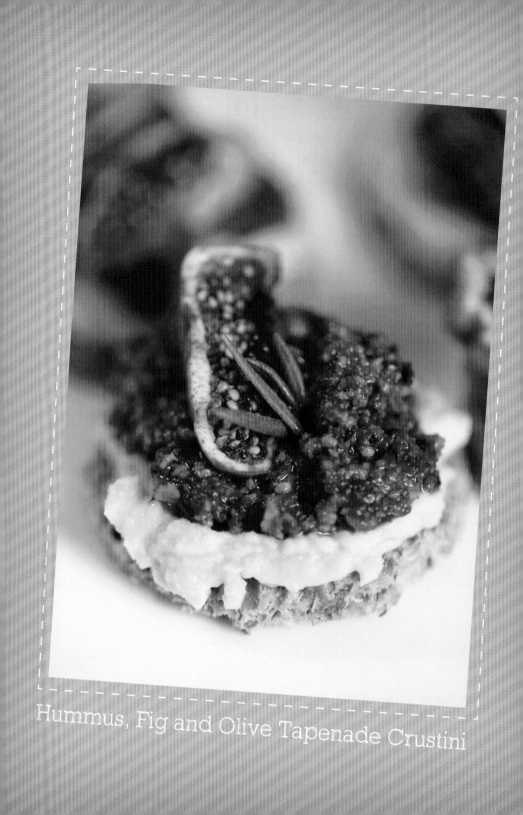

Hummus, Fig and Olive Tapenade Crustini

Hummus, Fig and Olive Tapenade Crustini

This tapenade makes an excellent canapé or spread for your fave wrap. Not only is it extremely heart-healthy – loaded in essential fatty acids and fibre, but it's also extremely delish! The figs add a nice touch of sweetness and are one of the most alkalizing and mineral rich foods around – plus extremely high in calcium, contributing to bone health.

FIG AND OLIVE TAPENADE:
- ½ cup dried figs
- ½ cup SaviSeed – Oh Natural
- 2 cups black Kalamata olives, pitted
- 2 tsp capers
- 1 tsp dried oregano
- 2 tbsp juice of freshly squeezed orange
- 1 tbsp Vega Antioxidant EFA Oil Blend
- freshly ground black pepper to taste
- 4 fresh figs, as garnish

Rehydrate dried figs in a bowl of warm water for about one hour until they are plump and tender. (Or to speed things up, bring water to a boil in a sauce pan then reduce to low heat. Add the figs and simmer for about 15 minutes.) Add SaviSeeds to food processor and pulse until ground. Remove from food processor and set aside. Once figs are rehydrated, give them a rough chop and pulse together with olives, capers, oregano, and freshly squeezed orange juice in food processor until finely chopped. Transfer mixture to mixing bowl, stir in Vega Antioxidant EFA Oil blend and season with pepper. Stir in ¾ of the ground SaviSeeds into tapenade. Set aside the rest as garnish for crustini.

Recipe continues on next page.

Hummus, Fig and Olive Tapenade Crustini Cont'd

HUMMUS:
- 3 cups chickpeas, cooked
- Juice of 1 lemon
- 2 cloves of garlic, minced
- ¼ cup water
- ¼ cup extra virgin olive oil
- 1½ tsp ground cumin
- ¼ tsp sea salt
- ¼ tsp cayenne

Place all ingredients in food processor or blender and blend until smooth. You may adjust water for desired level of creaminess.

TIP:
Try dipping a variety of raw seasonal veggies in hummus or use as a delicious and nutritious spread for you sandwiches and wraps.

SPROUTED GRAIN CRISPS:
- 4 slices of sprouted grain bread
- 2 tbsp extra virgin olive oil
- 1 medium garlic clove, minced
- 1 tbsp finely chopped rosemary

Preheat oven to 325°F. Using a rolling pin, flatten out each slice of sprouted grain bread until flat. Using a round cookie cutter, cut out round circle shapes of the bread. Stir olive oil with garlic. Lightly brush each round with garlic/olive oil mixture. Place on a baking sheet in a single layer. Lightly sprinkle chopped rosemary overtop. Bake for 15 to 20 minutes or until lightly golden and crisp. Let crisps cool on a wire cooling rack.

Once sprouted grain crisps are cool, first spread layer of Hummus, then dollop with Fig and Olive Tapenade and garnish with remaining ground SaviSeed and thin slice of fresh fig.

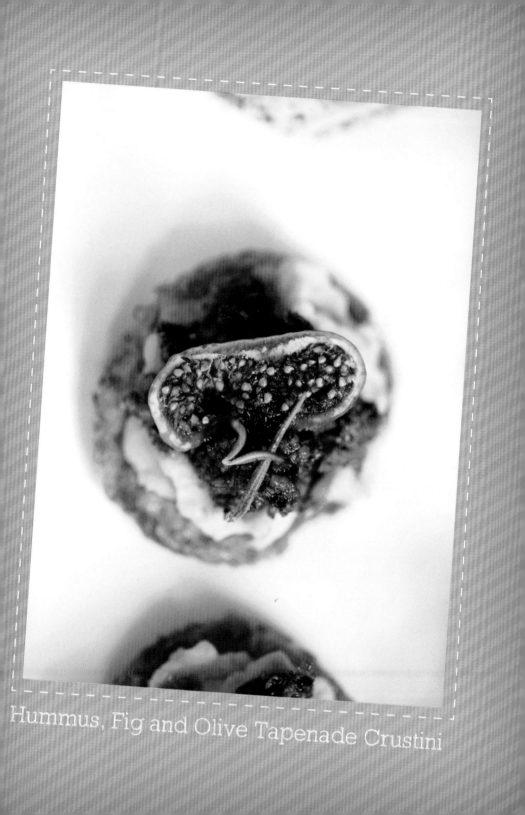

Hummus, Fig and Olive Tapenade Crustini

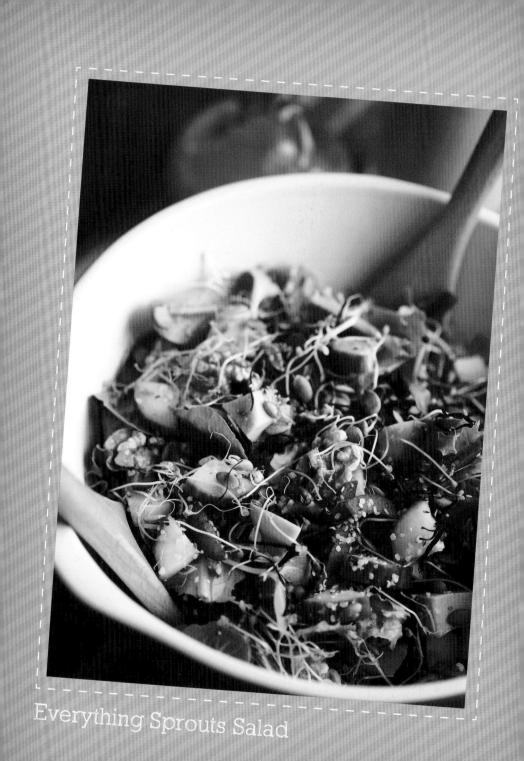

Everything Sprouts Salad

Everything Sprouts Salad

The ultimate nutrient-rich salad power-packed with chlorophyll, fibre, phytonutrients, trace minerals and vitamins.

SALAD:
- 2 cups sunflower sprouts
- 4 cups mixed greens
- ½ cup small sprouts, such as broccoli, alfalfa
- 1 ripe avocado, cubed
- ½ cucumber, chopped
- 1 red pepper, chopped
- ¼ cup arame, broken into pieces
- 2 tbsp raw pumpkin seeds
- 3 tbsp raw whole walnuts
- 2 tbsp hemp seeds
- ½ tsp kelp granules

Add all ingredients into a large bowl and drizzle with dressing of choice.
Makes 4–6 servings.

VINAIGRETTE DRESSING:
- ½ cup extra virgin olive oil
- ¼ cup balsamic vinegar or apple cider vinegar
- Juice of ½ lemon
- 1 tbsp dried oregano
- Sea salt and fresh black pepper to taste
- 1 tbsp stone ground Dijon mustard

Add all ingredients to bowl and whisk together. Optional: to make dressing extra creamy, whisk in 1–2 tbsp of hummus.

Recipe continues on next page.

HEMP AVOCADO DRESSING:

- 1 very ripe avocado
- ¼ cup hemp oil
- Juice from 1 lemon
- 2 tbsp fresh cilantro leaves, minced
- 2 tsp apple cider vinegar
- ¾ cup water
- Sea salt and fresh black pepper, to taste

Scoop avocado out of skin and place blender. Add hemp oil, lemon juice, cilantro, pepper, and vinegar. Blend well and thin with water, if necessary. Add sea salt and fresh black pepper to taste.

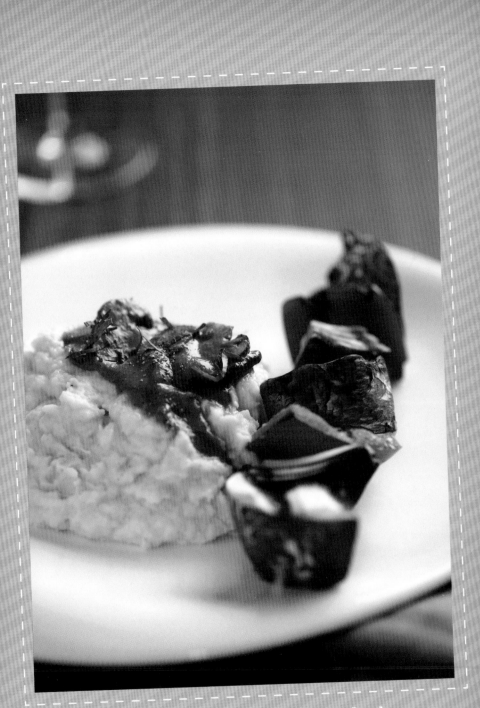

Portobello Kebabs with Garlic Mash
and Mo'shrooms

Portobello Kebabs with Garlic Mash & Mo'shrooms

Hail to the shroom! Who knew these tasty fungi stimulate your immune system, boost and regulate disease-fighting white blood cells so that they are ready to attack against whatever comes its way?

GARLIC MASH:
- 1 small cauliflower, cut into florets
- 1 parsnip, peeled and chopped
- 2 cloves garlic, minced
- ¼ cup extra virgin olive oil
- ¼ tsp sea salt
- ½ tsp ground cumin

Steam cauliflower and parsnip until tender, approximately 10 minutes. Add to blender with remaining ingredients and blend until smooth.

MUSHROOM GRAVY:
- 1 tbsp coconut oil
- 2 cloves garlic, minced
- 1 cup maitaki mushrooms, chopped
- 1 cup shiitake mushrooms, chopped
- 1 cup crimini mushrooms, chopped
- 1 cup button mushrooms, chopped
- ½ tsp ground chia seed
- 1 cup veggie stock or water
- Sea salt to taste

Heat coconut oil on medium heat. Add garlic and mushrooms and sautee until mushrooms have browned. Add half the mushroom mixture to blender and blend until smooth. Add ground chia and continue blending until well combined. Pour into bowl and stir-in remaining mushrooms.

KEBABS INGREDIENTS:
- ¼ cup extra virgin olive oil
- 2 garlic cloves, minced
- ½ tsp sea salt
- 2 Portobello mushrooms, cut into 1" pieces
- 2 red peppers, cut into 1" pieces
- 1 red onion, cut into 1" pieces

DIRECTIONS:
Preheat grill or barbeque and soak eight large wooden skewers in water for 20 minutes. In a small bowl, whisk together olive oil, garlic and sea salt; set aside. Thread a piece of Portobello mushrooms followed by a piece of red pepper and a chunk of red onion. Repeat until the skewer is full. Repeat threading the remaining vegetables onto the rest of the skewers. Brush skewers with olive oil and garlic marinade and grill, turning occasionally, until warmed through. Serve immediately with Garlic Mash and Mushroom Gravy. Serves four.

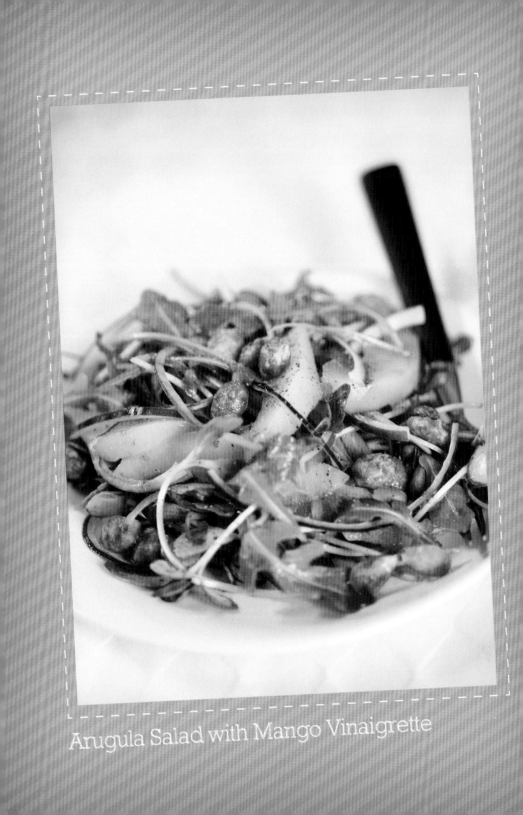

Arugula Salad with Mango Vinaigrette

Arugula Salad with Mango Vinaigrette

The health benefits of leafy greens are vast – packed with vitamins, minerals, fibre, chlorophyll and phytonutrients. Add sprouts and you can see that nutrition profile increase by as much as 100–600%!

DRESSING:
- ½ cup extra virgin olive oil
- ¼ cup balsamic vinegar
- 1 tbsp Vega Shake & Go Smoothie – Tropical Tango
- 1 tsp dried oregano
- Sea salt and fresh black pepper to taste

Whisk ingredients together well. Season with sea salt and black pepper to taste.

SALAD:
- 4 cups arugula
- 1 cup sunflower sprouts
- 1 poached pear, sliced
- ½ cup SaviSeed – Karmalized
- ½ red onion, sliced

Toss dressing with arugula and sunflower sprouts. Plate arugula and sunflower sprouts and top with pear, SaviSeed and red onion.

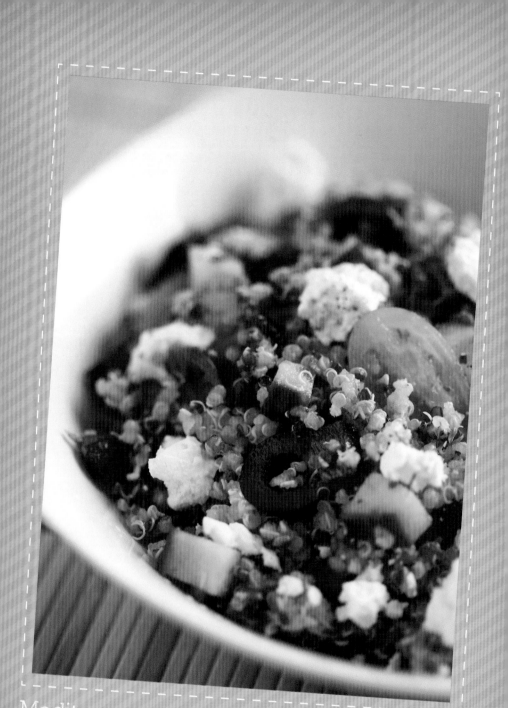

Mediterranean Quinoa Salad

Mediterranean Quinoa Salad

Quinoa is a definite staple in my kitchen! This simple salad using leftover quinoa is super fast and easy to make. Plus you get the benefit of energizing B vitamins, muscle-relaxing magnesium, and blood-sugar-balancing fibre. What's not to love?

- 2 cups cooked white quinoa
- 1 cup grape tomatoes, halved
- ½ cup cucumber, diced
- ½ cup black olives, pitted and chopped
- ½ red bell pepper, diced
- ¼ cup feta cheese, crumbled (optional)
- 3 tbsp extra virgin olive oil
- ½ tsp sea salt
- Pinch fresh ground black pepper
- 1 tsp dried oregano
- Juice of ¼ lemon

Add all ingredients to a bowl and mix well.

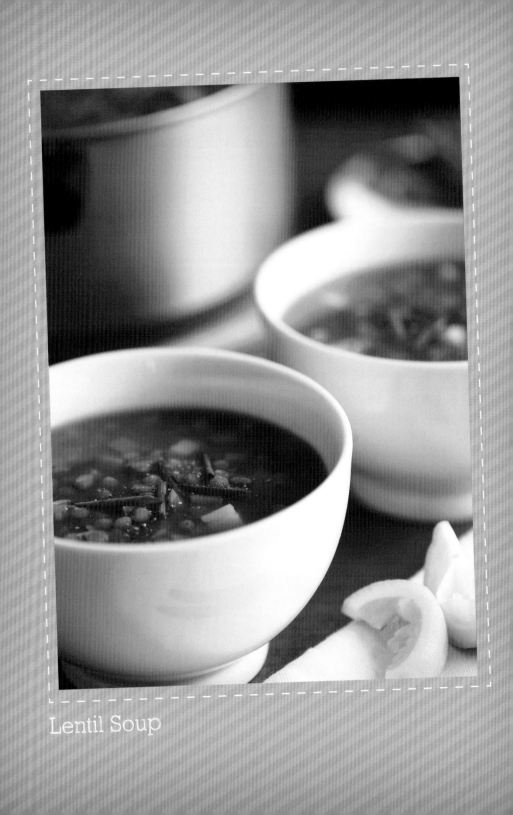

Lentil Soup

Lentil Soup

Lentils are packed with cholesterol-lowering, hunger-busting, blood sugar-balancing fibre, along with protein, tryptophan, which stimulates your 'happy' neurotransmitters, and iron, to boost energy. Adding red peppers to the soup helps to increase iron absorption due to high vitamin C content. Plus, this is my grandma's recipe, so it truly is the perfect comfort dish!

- 12 oz. or 1 ¾ cup dry brown or green lentils
- 1 large white onion, diced
- 1 green pepper, diced
- 1 celery stalk, diced
- 2 carrots, diced
- 6 cloves garlic, minced
- 2 medium tomato, crushed or ½ 15 oz. can or ¾ cup crushed tomatoes
- 1 small potato (Yukon gold or red potato) peeled and cut in quarters
- 1 tsp paprika
- 5 bay leafs
- ½ tsp dried oregano
- Sea salt and freshly ground black pepper to taste
- Juice from 1 lemon

Rinse lentils thoroughly. Cover with 4 cups water in small pot and bring to a boil. Once boiled, rinse lentils again and add to large pot filled with 8 cups water. Add onion, green pepper, celery, carrots, garlic, tomato, potato, paprika and bay leafs to pot and bring to a boil. Continue to boil until lentils become soft approximately 15–20 minutes. Remove potato from pot, cut into small cubes or mash with a fork and add back to pot. Reduce to a simmer and add oregano, salt and black pepper to taste.* Before serving remove bay leaves and stir in lemon juice. Makes about 3 litres. I love to store this recipe in single-serve containers in the freezer and grab when I need a meal!

OPTION:
Use pinch of cayenne instead of black pepper and 1 tsp kelp granules instead of sea salt for an added nutrition boost.

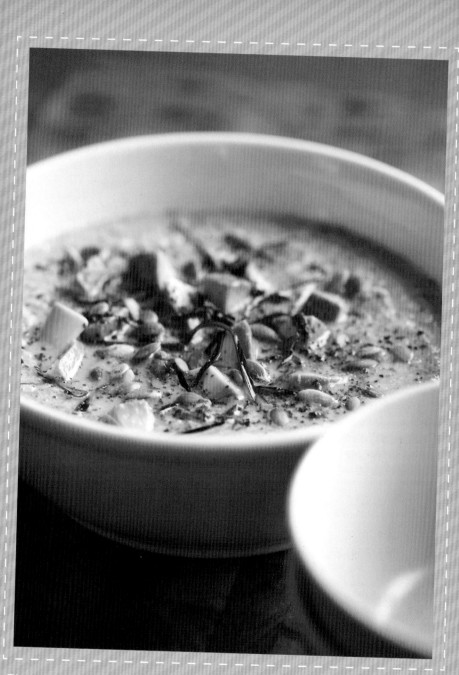

Creamy Brocolli Soup

Creamy Broccoli Soup

This is super quick and easy... and super creamy... without the cream! All ingredients are used raw, except for the steamed broccoli, which is required to help break down the cell wall and goitrogens if you have a sluggish thyroid.

SOUP:
- 1 head of broccoli, chopped into florets
- 2 stalks celery, chopped
- ½ small yellow onion, chopped
- 1 clove garlic, minced
- 1" piece fresh ginger, peeled and chopped
- Juice of ½ lemon
- 1 tsp dried oregano
- ½ tsp fresh ground black pepper
- Pinch sea salt
- ½ cup veggie stock or water
- 2 tbsp olive oil
- 1 avocado, diced (optional)

TOPPING:
- 2 tbsp pumpkin seeds
- ¼ avocado cubed into pieces
- ¼ cup arame, broken into pieces
- 1 tsp dulse flakes or kelp granules
- Pinch cayenne pepper

Steam broccoli until slightly tender, approximately three minutes. In meantime, add celery, onion, garlic, ginger, lemon juice, oregano, salt and black pepper to high-speed blender. Add the broccoli and ½ cup veggie stock or water. Blend until well combined. If soup seems too thick, adjust consistency with more veggie stock or water. Add olive oil and adjust seasoning with salt and black pepper to taste. Soak dried arame in water for 5–10 minutes and then rinse. Add soup to serving bowls and top with pumpkin seeds, avocado, arame, dulse or kelp and cayenne. Serves four.

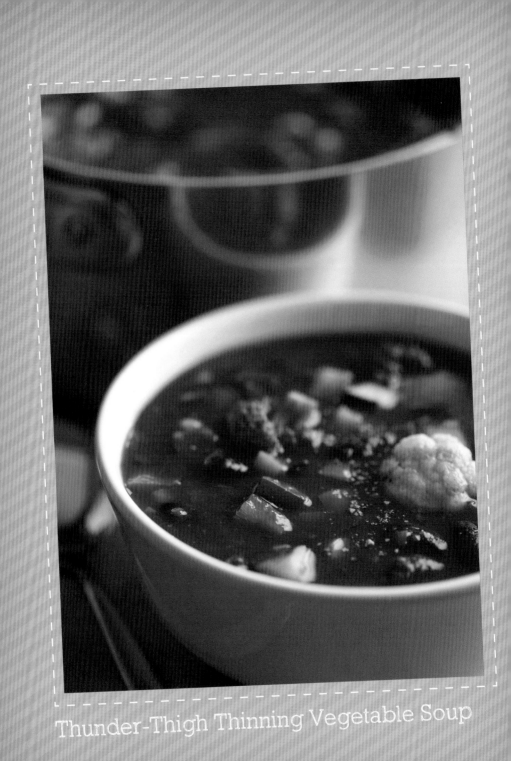

Thunder-Thigh Thinning Vegetable Soup

Thunder-Thigh Thinning Vegetable Soup

High nutrient and low calorie: a winning combo when you want to wave good bye to a couple pounds. This thigh-loving soup helps you achieve your weight loss goals, as it's high fibre and protein help keep you full for hours.

INGREDIENTS:
- 1 large white onion, diced
- 4–5 cloves garlic, minced
- 1 cup celery, diced
- 1 cup carrots, diced
- ¾ cup green peppers, chopped
- ¾ cup red peppers, chopped
- 4 medium tomatoes crushed (or 1-16 oz. can crushed tomatoes)
- 1 ½ cups broccoli florets
- 1 ½ cups cauliflower florets
- 1 cup zucchini, chopped
- 1 14 oz. can red kidney beans
- 1 tsp paprika
- ½ tsp dried oregano
- Salt and black pepper to taste

DIRECTIONS:
Fill a large pot with 6 cups water, add tomatoes, onion, celery, carrots, green pepper, red pepper and garlic and bring to boil. Continue to boil until veggies are soft, about 8 minutes. Then add broccoli, cauliflower, zucchini, kidney beans, paprika, oregano and a few grinds of fresh black pepper and continue to boil for another 5–10 minutes. Reduce to simmer and add a pinch of salt to taste. Ladle soup into bowls and serve with a few slices of sprouted grain bread on the side. This is another great soup to eat throughout the week or freeze for future meals!

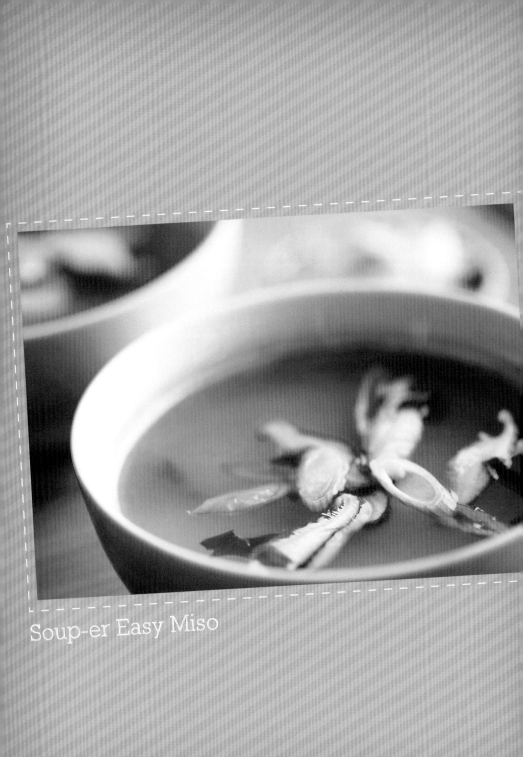

Soup-er Easy Miso

Soup-er Easy Miso

This soup is uber easy to make and does wonders for your digestive health AND immune system. Kiss belly-bloat buh-bye and make room for all those cancer-kicking cells!

- 4½ cups water
- ¼ cup yellow miso
- ¾ cups shiitake mushrooms
- ¼ cup wakame, broken in pieces
- 1 scallion, chopped

On high heat, add water to a pot and boil. Once water reaches a boil, stir in miso and remove from heat, until dissolved. Divide mushrooms, wakame and scallions among bowls. Ladle miso broth into bowls. Let sit for a few minutes and enjoy. Serves four.

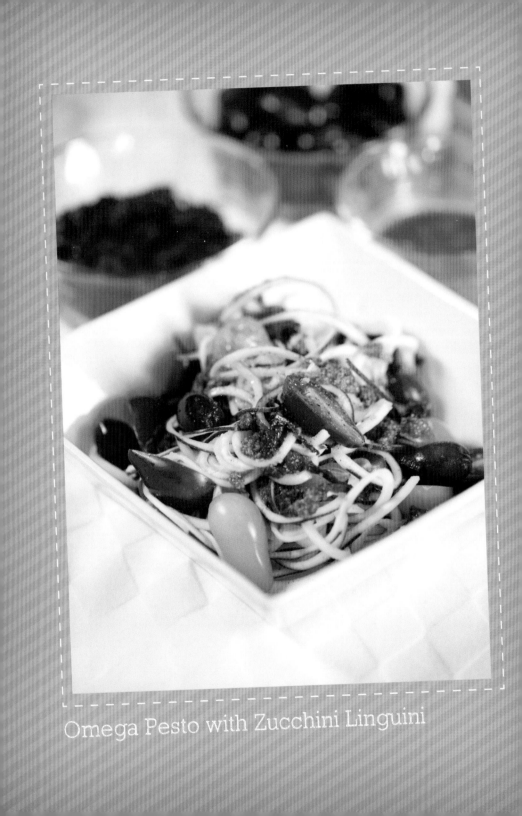

Omega Pesto with Zucchini Linguini

Omega Pesto with Zucchini Linguini

This pesto is loaded in Omega-3, protein and flavour! It goes great served on cooked quinoa, brown rice pasta, kelp noodles or zucchini linguini for a low-cal take!

PESTO:
- ½ cup SaviSeed – Oh Natural
- 2 tbsp hemp seeds
- 2 cups fresh basil
- 3 cloves garlic
- ½ cup extra virgin olive oil
- 1 tsp sea salt

Add all ingredients to food processor and process until well combined.

TOPPING:
- ½ pint cherry or grape tomatoes
- ½ cup black Kalamata olives
- ½ cup sundried tomatoes, chopped

ASSEMBLY:
Add 1–2 tbsp of pesto to 1 cup of cooked quinoa, pasta or zucchini linguini and mix until well combined. Top with tomatoes, olives and sundried tomatoes.

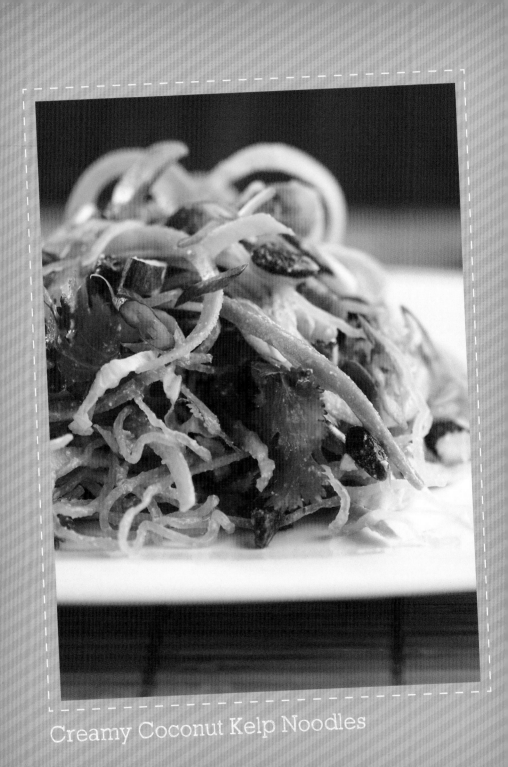

Creamy Coconut Kelp Noodles

Creamy Coconut Kelp Noodles

This dish is a healthy take on Pad Thai, only it's completely raw and loaded with ingredients to give your metabolism a kick into overdrive.

DRESSING:
- ¼ tsp toasted sesame oil
- ½ cup macadamia nuts
- ½ cup coconut milk
- 1 tbsp coconut oil
- 1" piece fresh ginger, minced
- 1 garlic clove, minced
- ½ tsp ground cumin
- 1 tbsp tamari
- ¼ tsp paprika
- ¼ tsp cayenne pepper
- 2 tbsp lime juice

Add all ingredients to high powder blender and blend until smooth.

NOODLES:
- ⅓ cup goji berries
- 1 bag kelp noodles
- 2 cups sunflower spouts
- 1 large carrot, julienned
- 2 scallions, thinly sliced
- 1 cup Napa cabbage, shredded
- 1 golden beet, sliced using a spiral slicer or julienned
- 1 cup fresh cilantro leaves
- ½ cup almonds, coarsely chopped

Rehydrate goji berries in 1 cup water for 10 minutes. In a large bowl, toss all ingredients together along with enough dressing to lightly coat noodles. Dish up and enjoy! Serves six.

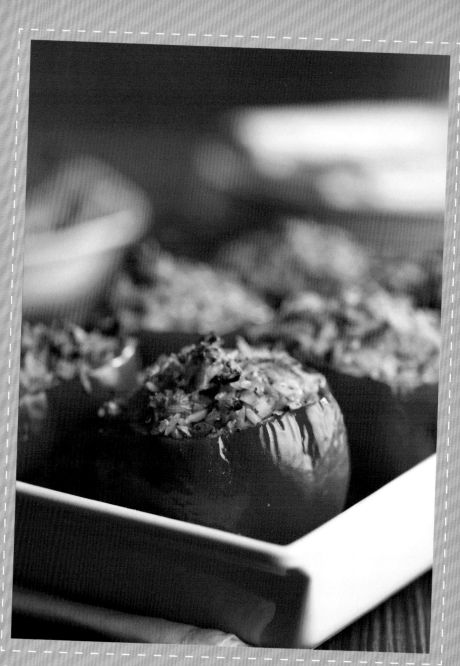

Stuffed Bell Peppers

Stuffed Bell Peppers

These take some time to make — mostly the chopping of vegetables — but if you have a food processor, it works wonders for this recipe! In addition, make this recipe in bulk and freeze individual servings for a great dinner or lunch any day of the week!

- 6 red pepper, with tops cut off and cored
- ¾ cup brown rice
- 1 onion, diced
- 2 cloves garlic, minced
- 1 zucchini, grated
- 1 large carrot, grated
- 1 celery stalk, diced
- 1 tsp dried thyme
- 1 tsp dried oregano
- ¼ tsp paprika
- ¼ tsp cayenne pepper
- 3 tbsp olive oil
- Sea salt and fresh ground black pepper to taste

Preheat oven to 350° F. Cut the tops off each pepper; clean out the stem portion and seeds. Stand the peppers upright in a casserole dish and set aside. Cook rice until partially cooked; about three-quarters of the way. Warm 1 tbsp olive oil in a large pan over medium heat. Add the onion and garlic and sauté for two minutes. Add zucchini, carrot, celery, rice and thyme, oregano, paprika and cayenne; sauté until veggies are tender, about 5 minutes. Stuff peppers full of the rice mixture. Pour ¼ cup water in the bottom of the casserole dish, so the peppers don't stick to the bottom while cooking. Drizzle 1–2 tbsp olive oil over peppers and season with sea salt and black pepper. Cover and bake for approximately 45–50 minutes. Serves six.

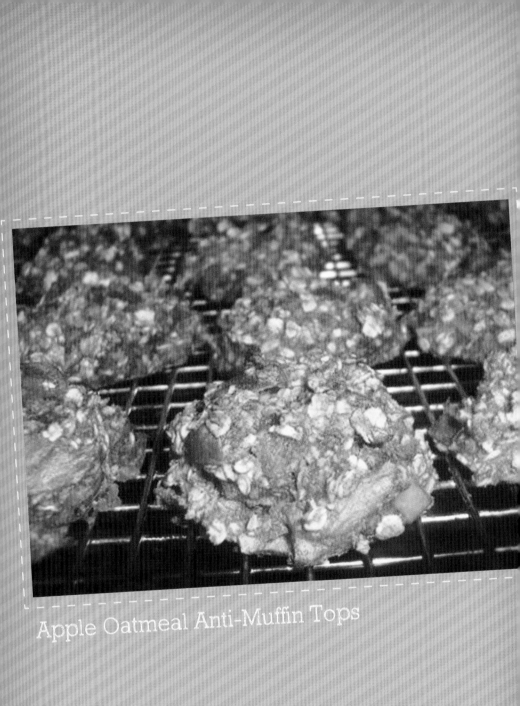

Apple Oatmeal Anti-Muffin Tops

Apple Oatmeal Anti-Muffin-Tops

These chewy cookies may taste like a muffin-top, but they can actually SHRINK your muffin-top! Apples and oats are a kick-ass heart-healthy, weight-loss combo. Both are super high in fibre helping to pull bad cholesterol from your body AND keep you full for longer periods of time, aiding in weight-loss.

- 5 apples peeled, cored and finely diced*
- ½ cup water
- 2 tsp ground cinnamon
- 3 cups old-fashioned rolled oats (uncooked)
- ½ cup apple butter
- ⅔ cup maple syrup
- Pinch sea salt

Pre-heat oven to 350°F. Place apples, water and cinnamon in small saucepan. Bring to a boil then simmer at medium-low heat till apples are soft, approximately 10 minutes. Remove pot from stove and stir in oats, then add apple butter, maple syrup and salt and mix well. Drop heaping tablespoons of batter onto parchment-lined cookie sheet and bake for 20–25 minutes. When done, carefully transfer cookies to wire racks and let cool.

*Baking apples: The best apples to use when baking are varieties that hold their shape, such as: Cortland, Empire, Granny Smith, Gala, Jonagold and Golden Delicious. Avoid varieties such as Pink Lady or Fuji that fall apart when baked or Red Delicious which tastes much better crunchy and raw.

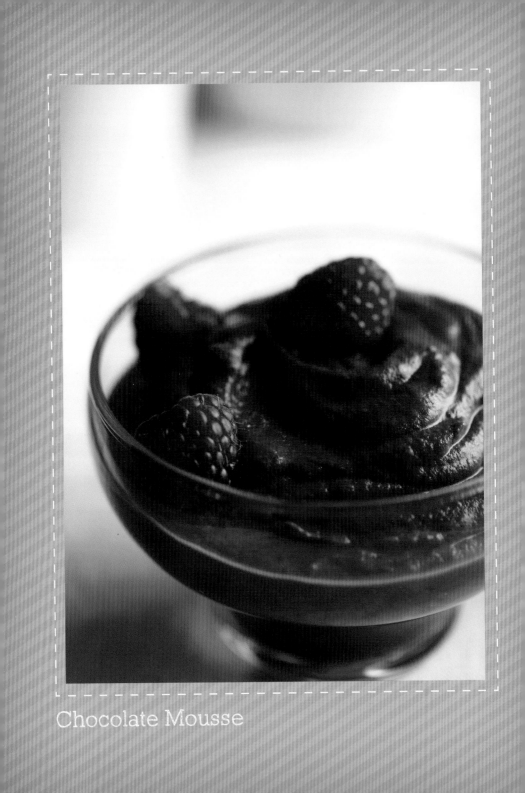

Chocolate Mousse

Chocolate Mousse

This mousse is so light, so airy, so decadent, and so HEALTHY! The secret ingredient? PUMPKIN! Yup! It's true. This guilt-free goodie helps to lower heart disease, prevent against cancer, and is great for expectant mums for its high folate content. You wouldn't even know! And oh so, so good.

- 2 cups cooked, pureed pumpkin
- ⅓ cup unsweetened cocoa powder
- ⅓ cup maple syrup
- ½ cup coconut oil, melted
- ½ tsp ground cinnamon
- ½ tsp vanilla extract

Add all ingredients to a bowl and mix well with a fork. That's it! Serves four.

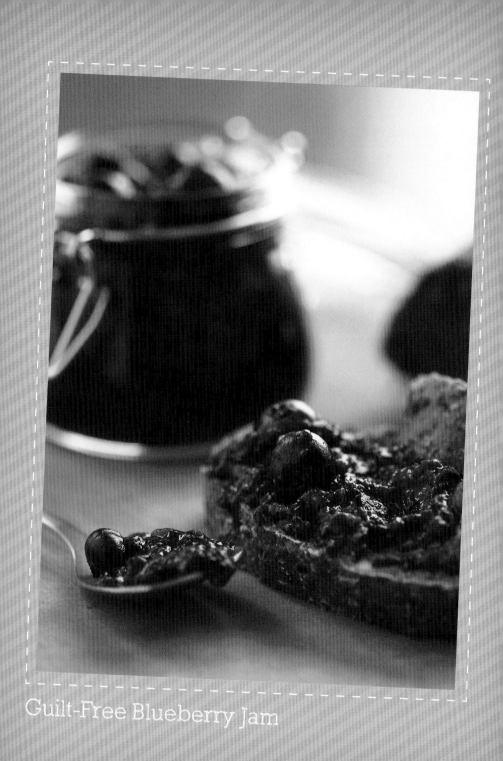

Guilt-Free Blueberry Jam

Guilt-Free Blueberry Jam

Free of additives, preservatives and added sugars, this recipe showcases the flavours of freshness, is super-simple to make AND can improve your complexion, lower cholesterol and reduce inflammation at the same time! The secret? Chia seeds!

- 1¼ cup fresh wild blueberries or other berries or fruits such as strawberries, peaches, fresh apricots, etc.
- ½ tsp vanilla extract
- 1 tsp coconut sugar (optional)
- 1 heaping tbsp ground chia seeds

Puree ¾ cup of berries in a food processor with vanilla and optional coconut sugar. Pour into bowl and stir in remaining whole berries and chia until well combined. Cover and refrigerate overnight. While you're sleeping – the chia will begin to gelatinize, turning your fresh berries into even MORE of an antioxidant-rich goodness! Serve on sprouted grain toast or use as topping for my Lemon Berry Tart (see recipe).

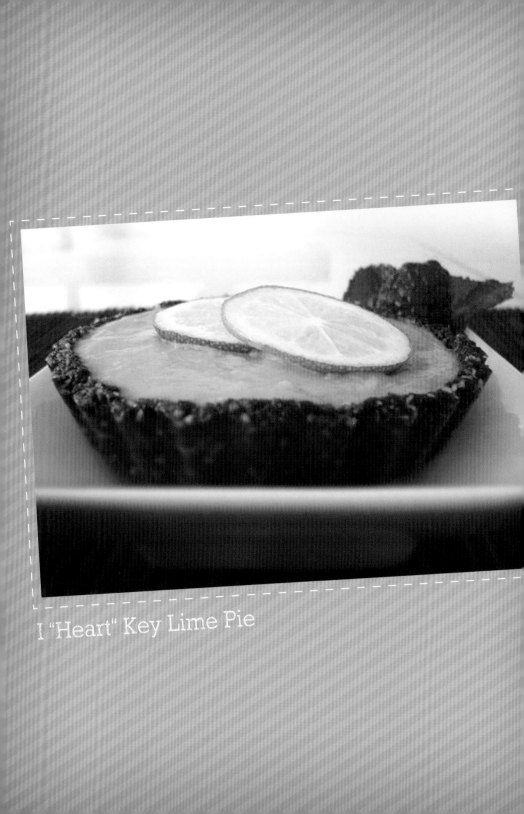

I "Heart" Key Lime Pie

I "Heart" Key Lime Pie

Not only will this melt-in-your-mouth, creamy, tangy and refreshing key lime pie steal your heart and have you falling in love, but while it's got it, it will also strengthen your heart! This smooth and tangy taste of sunshine can actually help lower cholesterol. Dig in — your heart (and tummy) will love you back!

CHOCOLATE MACAROON CRUST
- 1 cup pecans
- 1 cup raisins
- 1/3 cup unsweetened coconut flakes
- 3 tbsp cocoa powder
- 3 tbsp hemp seeds

Add all ingredients into food processor and mix until all ingredients are finely processed and start to stick together. Press mixture firmly into tart molds to form crust. Place in fridge while making the filling.

KEY LIME FILLING
- 1 large ripe avocado
- Juice of 2 limes
- Zest of ½ lime
- Juice of ½ lemon
- 1 tbsp extra virgin coconut oil
- 1/3 cup coconut nectar

Place all ingredients in food processor and blend until creamy and smooth. Pour into Chocolate Macaroon pie molds and refrigerate for at least one hour.

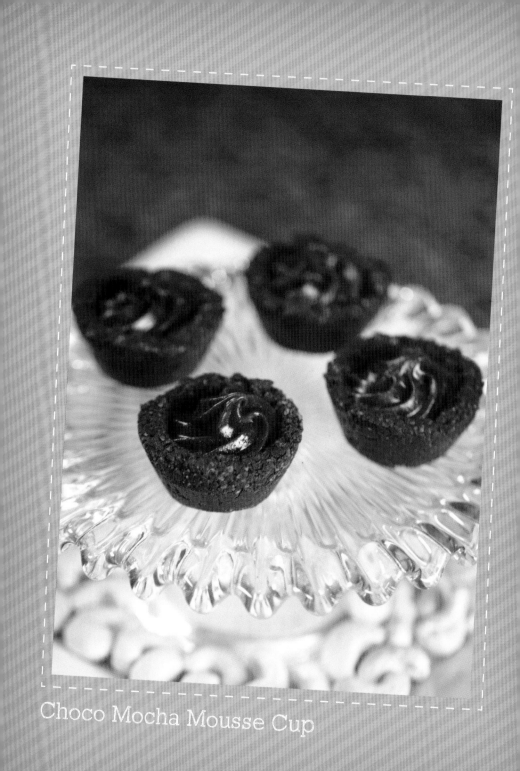

Choco Mocha Mousse Cup

Choco Mocha Mousse Cup

Decadent, indulgent and nutritious! This protein and fibre-rich dessert nourishes your body and wows your taste buds all at once.

CHOCO CUP:
- 1 MacaSure Chocolat bar
- 2 Vega Vibrancy Bars – Chocolate
- 1 tbsp raisins
- ½ tbsp cocoa powder

In double boiler, melt MacaSure Chocolate bar. While that's melting, combine all other ingredients in food processor and process well. Transfer mixture to bowl and stir in melted chocolate. Press into bottom and sides of a 4" spring-form pan or flexible mini muffin molds. Refrigerate.

CHOCO MOCHA MOUSSE:
- 2 cups raw cashews
- 2 tbsp Vega Shake & Go Smoothie – Choc-a-lot
- 1 shot fair-trade espresso
- 2 tbsp cocoa powder
- 3 tbsp coconut sugar
- ⅓ cup water
- 1 tsp vanilla extract
- 1 tbsp ground chia seeds

Add all ingredients – except ground chia – to a high power blender and slowly blend using the plunger to help mix the batter. You may need to add more water depending on consistency, but the batter should be thick. Finally, blend in the ground chia, incorporating well. Spoon out into Choco Cup. Refrigerate for at least two hours. Makes 10 mini tarts or one 6" tart.

BONUS:
The mousse can be eaten on its own as a rich, decadent dessert.

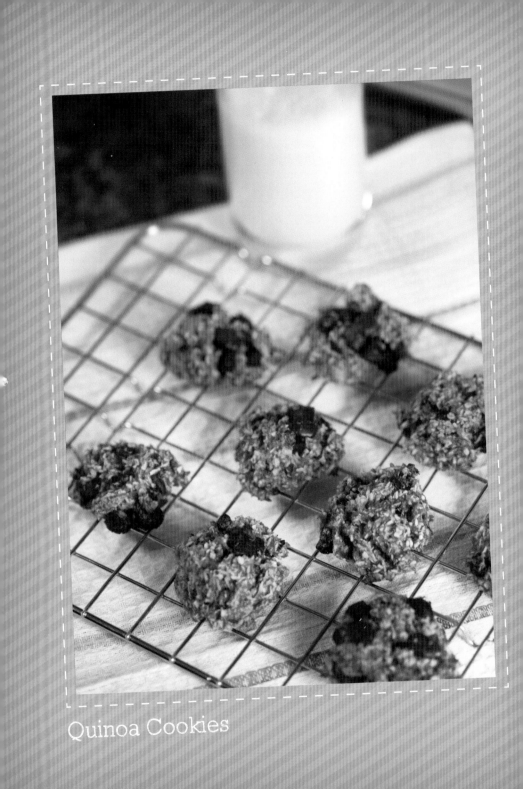

Quinoa Cookies

Quinoa Cookies

Once you have cooked quinoa on hand, you can eat it plain, throw it into shakes or smoothies as a thickening agent, use it as a cereal or substitute it for rice or pasta in your favourite dishes. My fave: cookies! Quinoa is loaded in nutrients and contains all essential amino acids making it a complete protein source.

- 4 large ripe bananas
- 1 tsp vanilla extract
- 1 cup cooked quinoa
- 1 cup uncooked quinoa flakes
- 1 cup unsweetened coconut flakes
- 2 tbsp MacaSure Powder
- ½ cup coconut sugar
- ½ cup dark, unsweetened chocolate chips OR MacaSure Chocolate Bar, broken in small pieces

Preheat oven to 380° F. In a large mixing bowl, mash bananas in bowl with a fork and add vanilla, quinoa, coconut, maca and coconut sugar. Mix until well combined. Stir in chocolate chips. Line baking sheet with parchment paper and drop heaping tablespoons of batter on to cooking sheet. Bake for 25–30 minutes – until cookie holds together. Remove from oven and let cool on a wire rack.

BONUS:
Replace the chocolate chips with ¼ cup of cacao powder to turn this recipe into chocolate quinoa cookies!

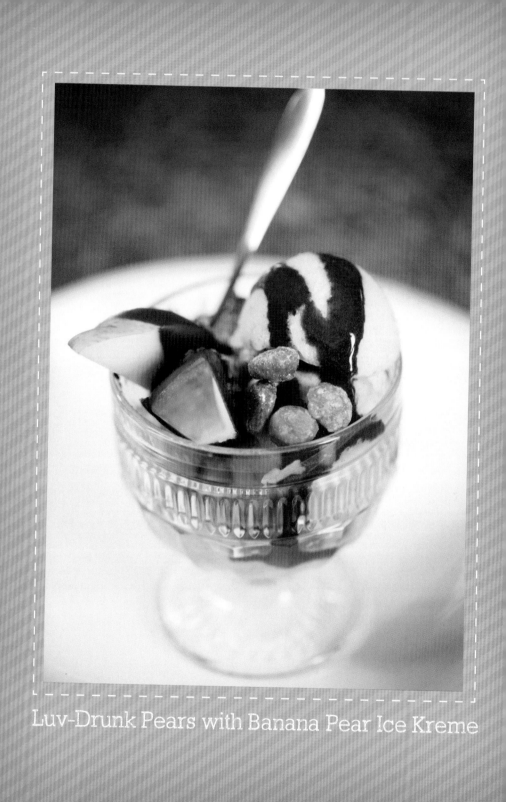

Luv-Drunk Pears with Banana Pear Ice Kreme

Luv-Drunk Pears with Banana Pear Ice Kreme

A sexy dessert featuring chocolate and maca – the combination of these two aphrodisiacs are sure to get you in the mood!

BANANA PEAR ICE KREME:
- 4 very ripe frozen bananas
- 1 ripe Bartlett pear, peeled and cored
- ½ tsp ground cinnamon
- Seeds from 1 vanilla bean pod

Blend all ingredients in high-speed blended until smooth. Transfer to a container and keep in the freezer until needed.

LUV-DRUNK PEARS:
- 4 MacaSure Chocolat bars
- 2 Bartlett pears
- Pinch Himalayan coarse sea salt

Melt MacaSure Chocolat in a double boiler. Cut pears into wedges. Dip pears half way into melted chocolate. Arrange on baking sheet lined with parchment paper. Sprinkle with salt crystals. Refrigerate until chocolate hardens.

COCOA-KISSED DRIZZLE:
- 2 tbsp yacon syrup
- 2 tsp cocoa powder
- ¼ tsp ginger powder

Scoop Banana Pear Ice Kreme into bowls, drizzle with Cocoa-Kissed Sauce and top with Luv-Drunk Pears.

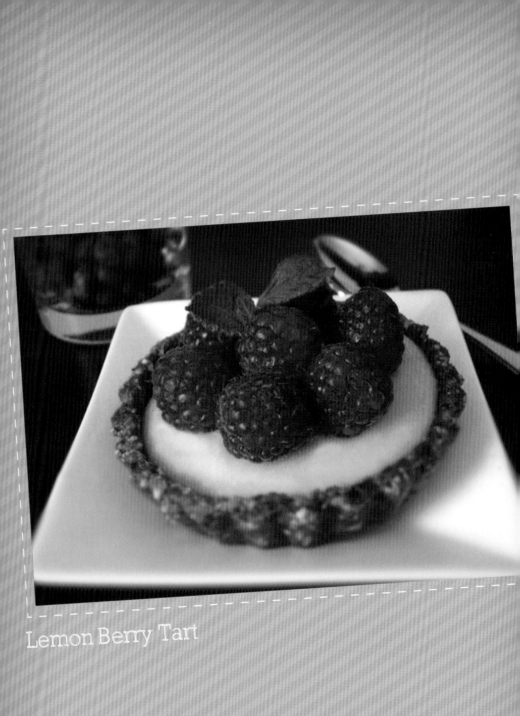

Lemon Berry Tart

Lemon Berry Tart

This tart is dairy-free, wheat-free, gluten-free, and soy-free. Yet, the tart, lemony cashew-cream filling is packed with vitamin C and protein aiding in muscle recovery. It's also loaded in antioxidants and minerals, such as magnesium, which help increase bone strength and promote relaxation. And the taste… absolutely delish!

TART SHELL:
- 1 cup pecans
- ½ cup raisins
- ½ cup dried cherries

Add pecans, raisins and cherries to food processor and process until finely chopped and mixture starts to stick together. Press mixture into a 6-inch spring form pan or mini flexible muffin forms and refrigerate at least 30 minutes.

LEMON FILLING:
- 1 ½ cups raw cashews
- Zest of 1 large lemon
- Juice of 1 large lemon
- Juice of ½ large orange
- 1 tsp vanilla
- 2 tbsp water
- ½ cup coconut palm nectar
- 1 tbsp ground chia

Add cashews, lemon juice and zest, orange juice, and vanilla to a high powered blender and slowly blend using the plunger or spatula to help mix the batter. Add coconut nectar and water to adjust sweetness and consistency. Blend until smooth; batter should be thick. Stir in ground chia. Spoon into prepared spring-form tart shell or muffin form tart shells. Top with fresh raspberries or Blueberry Jam (see recipe) and refrigerate for at least 3 hours.

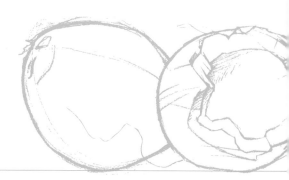

RESOURCES

SUPPLEMENTS

ChlorEssence: *chlorella*
My key staple for energy, immunity, beauty and just general wellness is chlorella.
I grab a handful of tablets a few times a day to keep me going. My favorite brand
is ChlorEssence; it's higher in chlorophyll, protein and CGF than any other brand
of chlorella.
www.chloressence.com

Vega: *plant-based supplements and foods*
When I'm travelling or on-the-go, I know I can easily get my nutrition needs
covered with Vega's line of plant-based beverages and bars. Vega Whole Food
Health Optimizer is an all-in-one meal replacement; kind of like an insurance policy
to ensure all your daily nutritional needs are covered. Also a big fan of the Vega
Antioxidant EFA Oil Blend. It makes a fantastic Omega 3-rich addition to salad
dressings, dips and sauces. Vega Smoothie Infusion adds a great nutritional boost
for smoothies and baked goodies.
www.myvega.com

MacaSure: *maca*
For my clients who are stressed, need more energy, have hormone imbalances,
or looking for a little boost in the love department, maca is my go-to supplement.
Great in smoothies or baked goods, but my personal fave is MacaSure Chocolat.
(Add with a glass of red wine — I'm in heaven!)
www.macasure.com

E3 Live: *AFA blue green algae*
www.e3live.com

Douglas Labs: *Relora*
www.douglaslabs.com

New chapter: *food-grade supplements*
Holy basil, Reishi mushrooms
www.newchapter.com

EBI Nutrition: *High potency fish oil*
www. ebinutrition.com

NutraSea: *fish oils*
www.ascentahealth.com

St. Francis Herb Farm: *supplements*
Passionflower, valerian, etc.
www.stfrancisherbfarm.com

AOR: *nutritional supplements*
I loove their vitamin B-complex and rhodiola.
www.aor.com

Metagenics: *nutritional supplements*
Love their probiotics and vitamin D drops!
www.metagenics.com

FOOD & DRINKS

SaviSeed: *sacha inchi seeds*
I always make sure to have healthy snacks on me at all times. One of my favorite
new snacks are sachi inchi seeds from Peru. They're super high in omega-3,
protein, fiber, antioxidants and tryptophan.
www.saviseed.com

Tonica: *kombucha*
The perfect elixir loaded in probiotics and enzymes. Just close your eyes and
pretend it's champagne!
www.thefairystonic.com

Food for Life Baking Co.: *sprouted-grain breads*
www.foodforlife.com

Tibetan Gold: *goji berries*
www.tibetangold.com

Manitoba Harvest: *hemp products*
www.manitobaharvest.com

Living Libations: *raw chocolate*
The most awesome raw chocolate bars, natural beauty/skin products and essential oils
www.livinglibations.com

Artisana: *raw nut butters*
www.premierorganics.org

Sunfood: *natural health foods*
www.sunfood.com

Ecoideas: *coconut palm sugar*
www.ecoideas.ca

Coconut Secret: *coconut nectar, coconut flour*
www.coconutsecret.com

Organic Traditions: *camu camu powder*
www.organictraditions.com

Cocoa camino: *organic, fair-trade chocolate*
www.cocoacamino.com

Navitas Naturals: *yacon syrup*
www.navitasnaturals.com

Nourish Tea: *various teas*
www.nourishtea.ca

Biji Tea: *holy basil tea*
www.florahealth.com

Zico: *coconut water*
www.zico.com

Manna Organics: *sprouted manna loaf*
www.mannaorganicbakery.com

Sea Tangle Noodle Company: *kelp noodles*
www.kelpnoodles.com

Maine Coast: *sea veggies, kelp and dulse granules*
www.seaveg.com

Live Organic Food Bar: *snacks*
Raw gluten-free granola, crackers (rosemary flax is my fave), snacks and cheesy kale chips.
www.livefoodbar.com

Two Girls Cooking: *raw crackers*
www.twogirlscooking.com

PRANA: *chia seeds and snacks*
www.pranana.com

Living Nutz: *soaked, sprouted and dehydrated nuts*
www.livingnutz.com

Green and Blacks: *organic chocolate and cocoa*
www.greenandblacks.com

Teatulia: *tea*
Tea bags are made out of 100% eucalyptus leaves.
www.teatulia.com

Upaya Naturals: *raw foods, nuts, cacao, snacks, supplements, and kitchen appliances.*
www.upayanaturals.com

SKIN CARE

Burt Bee's: *skin and beauty products*
www.burtsbees.com

Juice Beauty: *natural skin products*
www.juicebeauty.com

REFERENCES

Akhondzadeh, B. A., Moshiri, E., Noorbala, A. A., Jamshidi, A. H., Abbasi, S. H., & Akhondzadeh, S. (2007). Comparison of petal of Crocus sativus L. and fluoxetine in the treatment of depressed outpatients: A pilot double-blind randomized trial. Progress in neuro-psychopharmacology & biological psychiatry, 31(2), 439–442.

Akhondzadeh, S., Naghavi, H. R., Vazirian, M., Shayeganpour, A., Rashidi, H., & Khani, M. (2001). Passionflower in the treatment of generalized anxiety: A pilot double-blind randomized controlled trial with oxazepam. Journal of Clinical Pharmacy and Therapeutics, 26(5), 363–367.

Akhondzadeh, S., Fallah-Pour, H., Afkham, K., Jamshidi, A.-H., & Khalighi-Cigaroudi, F. (2004). BMC Complementary and Alternative Medicine, 4(1), 12.

Akhondzadehbasti, A., Moshiri, E., Noorbala, A., Jamshidi, A., Abbasi, S., & Akhondzadeh, S. (2007). Comparison of petal of Crocus sativus L. and fluoxetine in the treatment of depressed outpatients: A pilot double-blind randomized trial. Progress in Neuro-Psychopharmacology and Biological Psychiatry, 31(2), 439–442.

Stoll, A., Emanuel Severus, W., Freeman, M., Rueter, S., Zboyan, H., Diamond,E … (1999). Omega 3 Fatty Acids in Bipolar Disorder: A Preliminary Double-blind, Placebo-Controlled Trial. Archives of General Psychiatry, 56(5), 407–412.

Basu, A., Sanchez, K., Leyva, M. J., Wu, M., Betts, N. M., Aston, C. E., & Lyons, T. J. (2010). Green tea supplementation affects body weight, lipids, and lipid peroxidation in obese subjects with metabolic syndrome. Journal of the American College of Nutrition, 29(1), 31–40.

Bent, S., Padula, A., Moore, D., Patterson, M., & Mehling, W. (2006). Valerian for sleep: a systematic review and meta-analysis. The American journal of medicine, 119(12), 1005–1012.

Bhattacharyya, D., Sur, T. K., Jana, U., & Debnath, P. K. (2008). Controlled programmed trial of Ocimum sanctum leaf on generalized anxiety disorders. Nepal Medical College Journal, 10(3), 176–179.

Blask, D., Dauchy, R. T., & Sauer, L. (2005). Putting cancer to sleep at night: The neuroendocrine/circadian melatonin signal. Endocrine, 27(2), 179–188.

British Nutrition Foundations. (2001). Mood and Food. Retrieved from http://www.britishnutrition.org.uk/home.asp?siteId=43&sectionId=1436&subSubSectionId=1420&subSectionId=336&parentSection=302&which=5

Burkhardt, S., Tan, D. X., Manchester, L. C., Hardeland, R., & Reiter, R. J. (2001). Detection and quantification of the antioxidant melatonin in Montmorency and Balaton tart cherries (Prunus cerasus). Journal of agricultural and food chemistry, 49(10), 4898–4902.

Shepherd, C. (2003). Evening Primrose Oil: Lifting the Curse of PMS. Retrieved from http://www.evening-primrose-oil.com/pms.html

Chen, S., Oh, S.-R., Phung, S., Hur, G., Ye, J. J., Kwok, S. L., … (2006). Anti-Aromatase Activity of Phytochemicals in White Button Mushrooms (Agaricus bisporus). Cancer Research, 66(24), 12026–12034.

Chopra, D. (1995). Perfect digestion: The complete mind-body programme for overcoming disorders. New York: Crown Publishing.

Chow, N., Fretz, M., Hamburger, M., & Butterweck, V. (2010). Telemetry as a Tool to Measure Sedative Effects of a Valerian Root Extract and Its Single Constituents in Mice. Planta medica.

Connolly, D. A., McHugh, M. P., Padilla-Zakour, O. I., Carlson, L., & Sayers, S. P. (2006). Efficacy of a tart cherry juice blend in preventing the symptoms of muscle damage. British journal of sports medicine, 40(8), 679-83.

Costa, G. (2010). Lavoro a turni e rischio di cancro della mammella. Giornale italiano di medicina del lavoro ed ergonomia, 32(4), 454–457.

DeNoon, D. (2005). Drink More Diet Soda, Gain More Weight?: Overweight Risk Soars 41% With Each Daily Can of Diet Soft Drink. Retrieved from http://www. webmd.com/diet/news/20050613/drink-more-diet-soda-gain-more-weight

Dilworth, L. L., Omoruyi, F. O., Simon, O. R., Morrison, E. Y., & Asemota, H. N. (2005). The effect of phytic acid on the levels of blood glucose and some enzymes of carbohydrate and lipid metabolism. The West Indian medical journal, 54(2), 102–106.

Docherty, J. P., Sack, D. A., Roffman, M., Finch, M., & Komorowski, JR. (2005). A double-blind, placebo-controlled, exploratory trial of chromium picolinate in atypical depression: effect on carbohydrate craving. Journal of psychiatric practice, 11(5), 302–314.

Duan, P., & Wang, Z. M. (2002). [Clinical study on effect of Astragalus in efficacy enhancing and toxicity reducing of chemotherapy in patients of malignant tumor]. Zhongguo Zhong xi yi jie he za zhi Zhongguo Zhongxiyi jiehe zazhi, 22(7), 515–517.

Federation of American Societies for Experimental Biology. (2010). Honey as an antibiotic: Scientists identify a secret ingredient in honey that kills bacteria. Retrieved from http://www.sciencedaily.com /releases/2010/06/100630111037. htm#

Feily, A., & Namazi. (2009). Aloe vera in dermatology: A brief review. Giornale italiano di dermatologia e venereologia : organo ufficiale, 144(1), 85–91.

Grimes, M. (2009). Licorice Treats Peptic Ulcers and Helicobacter Pylori Infection. Retrieved from http://www.naturalnews.com/026711_ulcers_licorice_peptic. html

Hlebowicz, J., Darwiche, G., Bjorgell, O., & Almer, L. (2007). Effect of apple cider vinegar on delayed gastric emptying in patients with type 1 diabetes mellitus: A pilot study. BMC gastroenterology, 7, 46.

Howatson, G., McHugh, M. P., Hill, J. A., Brouner, J., Jewell, A. P., van Someren, K. A., ... (2010). Influence of tart cherry juice on indices of recovery following marathon running. Scandinavian journal of medicine & science in sports, 20(6), 843–852.

Jazayeri, S., Tehrani-Doost, M., Keshavarz, S. A., Hosseini, M., Djazayery, A., Amini, H., ... (2008). Comparison of therapeutic effects of omega-3 fatty acid eicosapentaenoic acid and fluoxetine, separately and in combination, in major depressive disorder. The Australian and New Zealand journal of psychiatry, 42(3), 192–198.

Wurtman, J. (2010). The Antidepressant Diet. Retrieved from http://www.psychologytoday.com/blog/the-antidepressant-diet/201008/you-can-prevent-pms-destroying-your-diet

Kang, S. Y., Seeram, N. P., Nair, M. G., & Bourquin, L. D. (2003). Tart cherry anthocyanins inhibit tumor development in Apc(Min) mice and reduce proliferation of human colon cancer cells. Cancer letters, 194(1), 13–19.

Auborn, K. (2003). Indole-3-Carbinol Is a Negative Regulator of Estrogen. The Journal of Nutrition, 133, 2470S-2475S.

Khan, A., Safdar, M., Ali, K. M. M., Khattak, K. N., & Anderson, R. A. (2003). Cinnamon improves glucose and lipids of people with type 2 diabetes. Diabetes care, 26(12), 3215–3218.

Kuehl, K. S., Perrier, E. T., Elliot, D. L., & Chesnutt, J. C. (2010). Efficacy of tart cherry juice in reducing muscle pain during running: A randomized controlled trial. Journal of the International Society of Sports Nutrition, 7, 17.

Larkworthy, W., & Holgate, P. F. (1975). Deglycyrrhizinized liquorice in the treatment of chronic duodenal ulcer. A retrospective endoscopic survey of 32 patients. The Practitioner, 215(1290), 787–792.

Lewith, G. T., Godfrey, A. D., & Prescott, P. (2005). A single-blinded, randomized pilot study evaluating the aroma of Lavandula augustifolia as a treatment for mild insomnia. Journal of alternative and complementary medicine, 11(4), 631–637.

Li, X. M., Ma, Y. L., & Liu, X. J. (2007). Effect of the Lycium barbarum polysaccharides on age-related oxidative stress in aged mice. Journal of ethnopharmacology, 111(3), 504–511.

Lin, P. Y., & Su, K. P. (2007). A meta-analytic review of double-blind, placebo-controlled trials of antidepressant efficacy of omega-3 fatty acids. The Journal of clinical psychiatry, 68(7), 1056–1061.

Ludvik, B., Neuffer, B., & Pacini, G. (2004). Efficacy of Ipomoea batatas (Caiapo) on diabetes control in type 2 diabetic subjects treated with diet. Diabetes care, 27(2), 436–440.

Maenthaisong, R., Chaiyakunapruk, N., Niruntraporn, S., & Kongkaew, C. (2007). The efficacy of aloe vera used for burn wound healing: a systematic review. Burns : journal of the International Society for Burn Injuries, 33(6), 713–718.

Brown, M. (2009). Evening Primrose Oil--For the Active Lifestyle. Retrieved from http://www.hhnews.com/epo.htm

Martin, J., Wang, Z. Q., Zhang, X. H., Wachtel, D., Volaufova, J., de Matthews, & Cefalu, W. T. (2006). Chromium picolinate supplementation attenuates body weight gain and increases insulin sensitivity in subjects with type 2 diabetes. Diabetes care, 29(8), 1826–1832.

Takikawa, M. (2010). Dietary Anthocyanin-Rich Bilberry Extract Ameliorates Hyperglycemia and Insulin Sensitivity via Activation of AMP-Activated Protein Kinase in Diabetic Mice. The Journal of Nutrition, 140(3), 527.

Murray, M. T. (1995). The healing power of herbs: The enlightened person's guide to the wonders of medicinal plants. Rocklin, CA: Prima Pub.

Turner, N. (2011). Four Keys to Kick PMS. Retrieved from http://www.truestarhealth.com/members/archives.asp?content=14ml3p1a97

Noorbala, A., Akhondzadeh, S., Tahmacebipour, N., & Jamshidi, A. (2005). Hydro-alcoholic extract of L. versus fluoxetine in the treatment of mild to moderate depression: A double-blind, randomized pilot trial. Journal of Ethnopharmacology, 97(2), 281–284.

Oi, Y., Imafuku, M., Shishido, C., Kominato, Y., Nishimura, S., & Iwai, K. (2001). Garlic supplementation increases testicular testosterone and decreases plasma corticosterone in rats fed a high protein diet. The Journal of nutrition, 131(8), 2150–2156.

Ozgoli, G., Goli, M., & Simbar, M. (2009). Effects of ginger capsules on pregnancy, nausea, and vomiting. Journal of alternative and complementary medicine 15(3), 243–246.

Patel, S. R., Malhotra, A., White, D. P., Gottlieb, D. J., & Hu, F. B. (2006). Association between Reduced Sleep and Weight Gain in Women. American Journal of Epidemiology, 164(10), 947–954.

Pigeon, W. R., Carr, M., Gorman, C., & Perlis, M. L. (2010). Effects of a tart cherry juice beverage on the sleep of older adults with insomnia: A pilot study. Journal of medicinal food, 13(3), 579–583.

Pongrojpaw, D., Somprasit, C., & Chanthasenanont, A. (2007). A randomized comparison of ginger and dimenhydrinate in the treatment of nausea and vomiting in pregnancy. Journal of the Medical Association of Thailand, 90(9), 1703–1709.

Psychology Today. (2003). Vitamin C: Stress Buster.Retrieved from http://www. psychologytoday.com/articles/200304/vitamin-c-stress-buster

Qi, F., Li, A., Inagaki, Y., Gao, J., Li, J., Kokudo, N., ... (2010). Chinese herbal medicines as adjuvant treatment during chemo- or radio-therapy for cancer. Bioscience trends, 4(6), 297–307.

Ried, K., Sullivan, T., Fakler, P., Frank, O. R., & Stocks, N. P. (2010). Does chocolate reduce blood pressure? A meta-analysis. BMC Medicine, 8(1), 39.

Pawlosky, R. (2001). Physiological compartmental analysis of alpha-linolenic acid metabolism in adult humans. The Journal of Lipid Research, 42, 1257–1265.

Erickson, R. (2010). Good Foods to Alleviate Menstrual Cramps. Retrieved from http://www.livestrong.com/article/94790-good-foods-alleviate-menstrual-cramps/

Sephton, S., & Spiegel, D. (2003). Circadian disruption in cancer: A neuroendocrine-immune pathway from stress to disease? Brain, behavior, and immunity, 17(5), 321–328.

Snitker, S., Fujishima, Y., Shen, H., Ott, S., Pi-Sunyer, X., Furuhata, Y., ... (2009). Effects of novel capsinoid treatment on fatness and energy metabolism in humans: Possible pharmacogenetic implications. The American journal of clinical nutrition, 89(1), 45–50.

Somerfield, S. D. (1991). Honey and healing. Journal of the Royal Society of Medicine, 84(3), 179.

Srinivasan, V., Spence, D. W., Pandi-Perumal, SR, Trakht, I., & Cardinali, D. P. (2008). Therapeutic actions of melatonin in cancer: Possible mechanisms. Integrative cancer therapies, 7(3), 189–203.

Swithers, S. E., & Davidson, T. L. (2008). A role for sweet taste: Calorie predictive relations in energy regulation by rats. Behavioral neuroscience, 122(1), 161–173.

Ma, T. (2011). What Does Fiber Do To Help Ease PMS? Retrieved from http://ezinearticles.com/?What-Does-Fiber-Do-To-Help-Ease-PMS?&id=1010265

Traustadottir, T., Davies, S. S., Stock, A. A., Su, Y., Heward, C. B., Roberts, L. 2., & Harman, S. M. (2009). Tart cherry juice decreases oxidative stress in healthy older men and women. The Journal of nutrition, 139(10), 1896–1900.

Wang, Y., Han, T., Zhu, Y., Zheng, C. J., Ming, Q. L., Rahman, K., & Qin, L. P. (2010). Antidepressant properties of bioactive fractions from the extract of Crocus sativus L. Journal of natural medicines, 64(1), 24–30. 6

Sansom, W. (2005). New analysis suggests 'diet soda paradox' – less sugar, more weight. Retrieved from http://www.uthscsa.edu/hscnews/singleformat2.asp?newID=1539

Zhang, Y., Vareed, S. K., & Nair, M. G. (2005). Human tumor cell growth inhibition by nontoxic anthocyanidins, the pigments in fruits and vegetables. Life sciences, 76(13), 1465–1472.